Manual on

Art of Labour

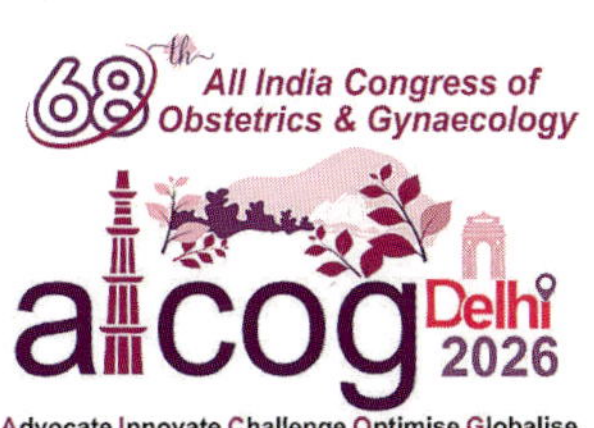

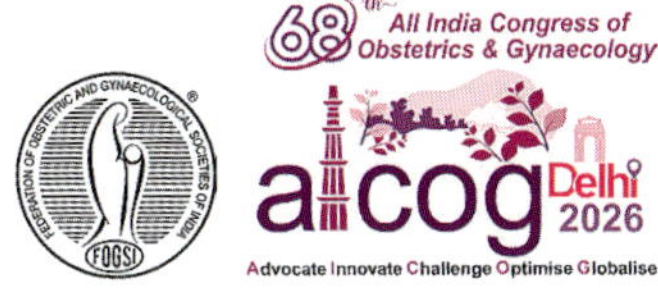

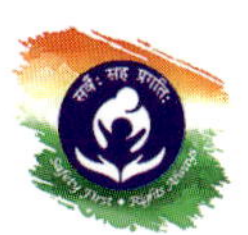
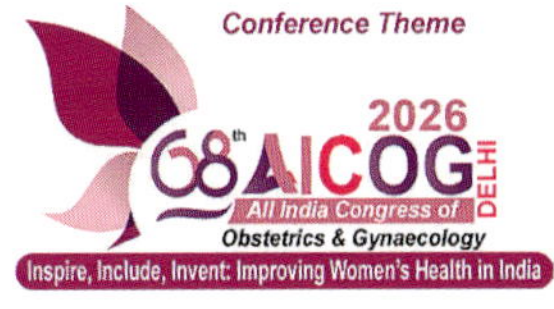

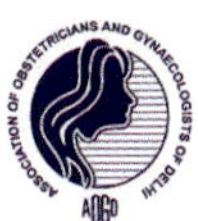

Manual on
Art of Labour

Series Editors

Ashok Kumar
MD PhD
Director–Professor
Department of Obstetrics and Gynecology
Atal Bihari Vajpayee Institute of Medical Sciences
and Dr Ram Manohar Lohia Hospital
New Delhi, India

Madhavi M Gupta
MS
Director–Professor
Department of Obstetrics and Gynecology
Maulana Azad Medical College and Lok Nayak Hospital
New Delhi, India

K Aparna Sharma
MBBS MD
Professor
Department of Obstetrics and Gynecology
All India Institute of Medical Sciences
New Delhi, India

Editors

Kanchan Sharma
Kamna Datta
Anita Sabherwal Anand
Gunjan Rai
Vinita Singh

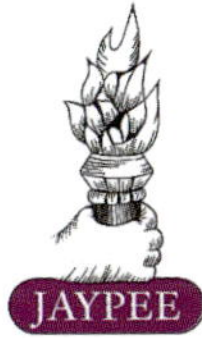

JAYPEE BROTHERS MEDICAL PUBLISHERS
The Health Sciences Publisher
New Delhi | London

Message from Series Editors

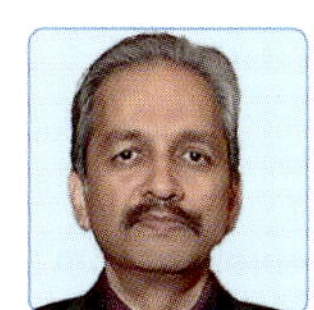

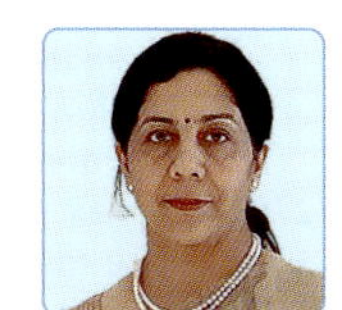

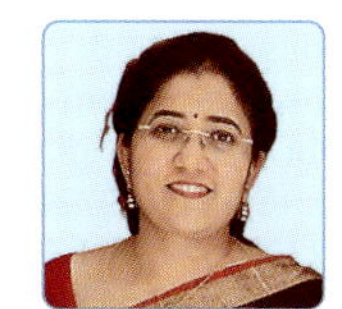

Ashok Kumar
Organizing Chairperson
AICOG-2026
New Delhi

Madhavi M Gupta
Organizing Secretary
AICOG-2026
New Delhi

K Aparna Sharma
Organizing Secretary
AICOG-2026
New Delhi

It is after 18 long years that the 68th AICOG is being held in New Delhi. It is a pleasure to welcome you all.

The Organizing Team have poured their heart and soul into curating an academic program which one will feel a loss if missed. The scientific sessions include both national and international faculty who are stalwarts in their fields. There are 18 workshops with 8 full-day and 5 each in the pre-lunch and post-lunch time.

On this occasion, the workshop faculty, have gone that extra mile to publish the workshop manual for eight workshops. This includes all recent scientific evidence and clinical management guidelines. These manuals will serve as a go-to evidence-based resource in your day-to-day clinical practice. We look forward to receiving your valuable feedback.

We acknowledge the hard work put in by all the editors, co-editors, and the authors, who, in spite of busy schedules and time constraints, have contributed immensely.

We would also like to thank M/s Jaypee Brothers Medical Publishers (P) Ltd, New Delhi, India, for partnering with us.

We sincerely hope that you will enjoy reading these manuals, find this manual useful, and treasure it for future use in your practical work.

We take this opportunity to wish you a memorable time during your stay in New Delhi.

Warm Regards

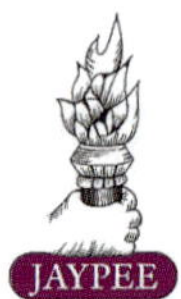

Jaypee Brothers Medical Publishers (P) Ltd

Headquarters
EMCA House, 23/23-B
Ansari Road, Daryaganj
New Delhi 110 002, India
Landline: +91-11-23272143, +91-11-23272703
+91-11-23282021, +91-11-23245672
e-mail: jaypee@jaypeebrothers.com

Corporate Office
4838/24, Ansari Road, Daryaganj
New Delhi 110 002, India
Phone: +91-11-43574357
Fax: +91-11-43574314
e-mail: jaypee@jaypeebrothers.com

Overseas Office
JP Medical Ltd.
83, Victoria Street, London
SW1H 0HW (UK)
Phone: +44-20 3170 8910
e-mail: info@jpmedpub.com

EU GPSR Authorised Representative
Logos Europe, 9 rue Nicolas Poussin
17000, La Rochelle, France
Phone: +33 (0) 6 67 93 73 78
e-mail: contact@logoseurope.eu

Website: www.jaypeebrothers.com
Website: www.jaypeedigital.com

Inquiries for bulk sales may be solicited at: jaypee@jaypeebrothers.com

Manual on Art of Labour

First Edition: **2026**

ISBN: 978-93-7545-897-5

Printed at: Samrat Offset Pvt. Ltd.

Contributors

Ajith S MD DGO DNB MRCOG FRCOG
Additional Professor
Department of Obstetrics and Gynecology
Government Medical College
Kannur, Kerela, India

Bharti Wadhwa MBBS MD FICA
Director and Professor
Department of Anesthesia
Maulana Azad Medical College
New Delhi, India

Chinmay Umarji
DGO MRCP (Ireland) MRCOG (London)
Fellowship in Fetal Medicine
Consultant
Sahyadri Superspeciality Hospitals
Consultant Umarji Hospitals
In-charge, Fetal Medicine Unit
BJ Medical college and
Sassoon General Hospital
Secretary (2022–2024) SFM Greater Pune Chapter
President elect SFM Greater Pune ChapTer

Jayasree Sundar
DGO (CAL) MRCOG (UK) RCOG (UK) FICOG FICMCH PGDMLS
Director
Madhukar Rainbow Children's Hospital
and BirthRight by Rainbow
New Delh, India

Jyoti Ramesh Chandran
MBBS MSFICOG IMS Diploma Urogynae
Professor and Head
Goverment Medical College
Kozhikode, Kerala, India

Jyotsna Suri
MD FICOG FRCOG (Hon)
Professor
Unit Head and In-charge
Obstetric Critical Care, Obstetrics and Gynecology
Vardhman Mahavir Medical College
and Safdarjung Hospital
New Delhi, India

Kanchan Sharma
MBBS MS FICOG FICMCH
IVF Specialist
Department of Obstetrics and Gynecology
Coordinator and Speaker of
Labour Workshop in AICOG
Chairperson
NCD Committee FOGSI

Mausumi De Banerjee
MBBS DGO DNB (Gyne & Obs) MNAMS FICOG FIAOG
Consultant Gynecologist
and Obstetrician
Kolkata, West Bengal, India
President BOGS (2023–2024)
Vice President IMA Calcutta (2021–2023)

Poonam Varma Shivkumar
MBBS MD
Director, Professor
(Obstetrics and Gynecology) and
Medical Superintendent
Kasturba Health Society
Mahatma Gandhi Institute of
Medical Sciences
Wardha, Maharashtra, India

Saburi Kulkarni
MBBS MS DNB (Obstetrics and Gynecology)
Junior Consultant
Umarji Mother and Child Care Hospital
Pune, Maharashtra, India

Sheela V Mane
MBBS MD FICOG FRCOG FICMCH
ICOG Chair 2026 and
Professor (Obstetrics and Gynecology)
Department of Family and Welfare
Government of Karnataka
KC General Hospital
Bengaluru, Karnataka, India

Preface

Labour is not merely a physiological event—it is a dynamic, time-sensitive process where science, skill, and judgment converge. Each contraction carries both promise and risk, and every decision made in the labour room has the potential to shape two lives. The *Art of Labour* lies in recognizing that while protocols guide us, outcomes are ultimately determined by anticipation, vigilance, and timely, thoughtful intervention.

This workshop has been conceived to bridge the space between textbook knowledge and bedside wisdom. The *Art of Labour* emphasizes that normal labour is not synonymous with passive observation, nor is intervention a sign of failure. Instead, excellence in intrapartum care demands continuous assessment, early recognition of deviation from normal, and decisive action taken with clarity and confidence.

The manual and deliberations within this workshop focus on real-world labour room challenges—interpreting progress, identifying early warning signs of maternal or fetal compromise, preventing avoidable morbidity, and responding effectively when labour veers off its expected course. Equal importance is given to communication, team coordination, and documentation, recognizing that safe labour care is a collective responsibility.

This initiative is designed to sharpen clinical acumen and reinforce structured, evidence-based approaches while respecting the individuality of each labouring woman. From peripheral setups to advanced tertiary centers, the principles discussed here are adaptable, practical, and rooted inpatient safety.

As obstetricians, we are custodians of one of the most critical transitions in human life. Mastery of labour is not achieved by intervention alone, but by knowing *when not to intervene, when to wait*, and *when to act without delay*.

It is my sincere hope that this workshop will enhance confidence, refine judgment, and inspire reflective practice—so that every birth is guided not just by competence, but by wisdom.

***Editors:* Kanchan Sharma, Kamna Datta,**
Anita Sabherwal Anand, Gunjan Rai, Vinita Singh

Contents

1 CHAPTER

Modern Labor Room Setup and Preparing Women for Labor

Poonam Varma Shivkumar

INTRODUCTION

Labor is a process which carries too many emotions together and the labor room experience has a major impact on not only mother and baby but also the family. The good experience in labor is a collaborative effort of women and the health providers, and it is also comprehensive as a successful labor depends on antenatal management also. In the present era when we are talking about Respectful maternity care and pregnant women rights in labor there are several changing trends in the labor management. Changing trends in labor management are dominated by technology (AI, data analytics, HR tech), flexibility (remote/hybrid work becoming standard), a focus on the pregnant women well-being and a shift towards skills-based development (upskilling/reskilling for digital/human skills) to have the best maternal and fetal outcomes. Key shifts include data-driven decisions, personalized laboring women journeys, integrating and promoting collaborative care and evolving good practice decisions for the modern laboring women with best quality.

COMPONENTS REQUIRED FOR SATISFYING LABOR EXPERIENCE

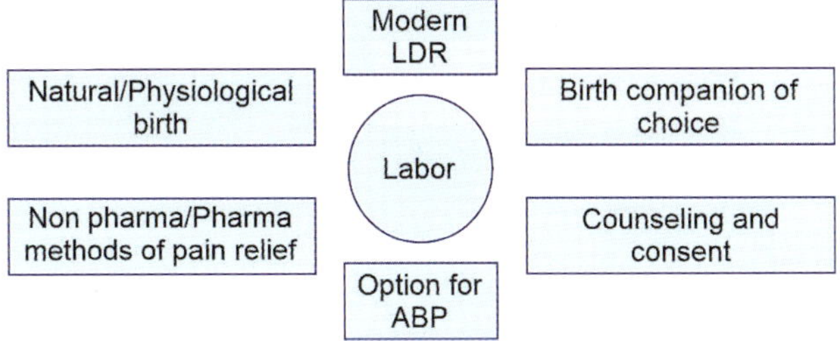

MODERN LABOR ROOM

Presently the Government of India recommends labor rooms with labor-delivery recovery (LDR) room concept (a pregnant woman spends the duration of labor, delivery, and 4 hours postpartum in the same bed) as they critically monitor women as compared to the conventional labor rooms (a pregnant woman is admitted to labor room only at or near full dilation of cervix and is shifted to the postpartum ward after 2 hours).

Such LDRs are designed to have labor cubicles with washroom and toilet in between, with privacy, each cubicle equipped with all necessary gadgets for alternative birthing, nonpharmacological methods of pain relief and labor trays for normal births. So, a modern labor room is a well-equipped, aseptic, and mother-friendly area designed to provide safe, respectful, and efficient care during labor, delivery, and the immediate postpartum period.

The two LDRs very close to each other separated by just one door are:

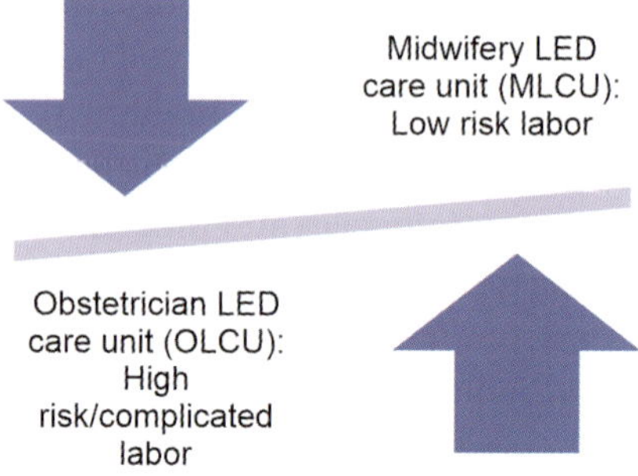

The ideal labor room layout proposed is as follows:

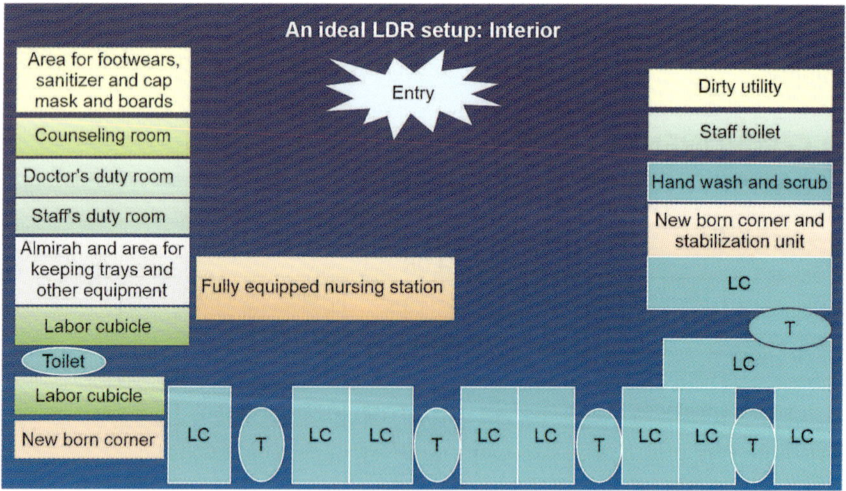

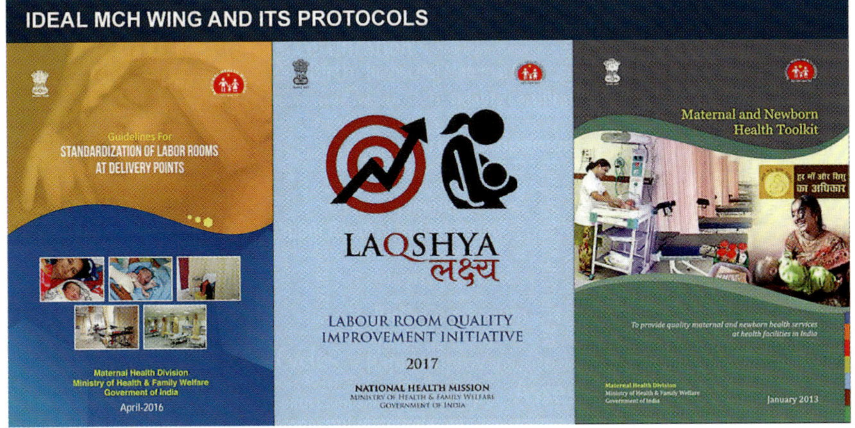

Objectives of LDR

- Ensure safe and natural/physiological delivery for mother and baby
- Reduce maternal and neonatal morbidity and mortality
- Provide privacy, comfort, emotional support , dignity and other rights
- Enable early detection and management of complications
- Provides supportive environment
- Provides appropriate maternal and fetal monitoring specially digitalized one
- Provides great birthing experience with baby mother family concept

Features of a modern labor room

- Clean, well-ventilated, and well-lit
- Maintains aseptic technique
- Ensures privacy (curtains/screens)
- Allows presence of a birth companion
- Equipped for normal and emergency deliveries

Essential Areas—Reception/assessment area, Obstetric triage, MLCU, OLCU, Newborn care corner, Post-delivery observation area

Essential Equipment—Delivery table/bed, Fetal monitoring devices, Stethoscope , fetoscope/Doppler/CTG, Sterile delivery instruments—Delivery tray, Oxygen, gas and Suction apparatus, Neonatal resuscitation equipment, Alternative birthing props—Birthing balls, mat, bean ball, birthing chair, hydrolabor tubs with system, aroma therapy, cold and hot packs etc, Emergency drugs (oxytocin, magnesium sulfate, etc.)

Human resource—Obstetricians,Staff nurse/midwife, Pediatrician/ neonatologist (on call), Anesthetist (if required)

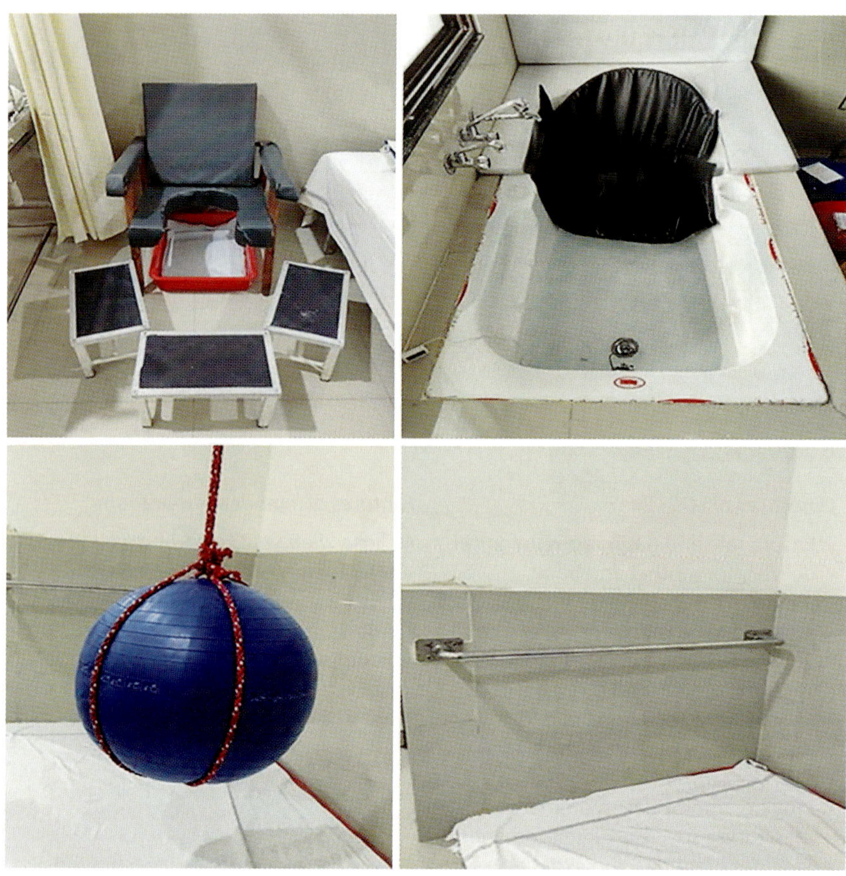

PREPARING WOMEN FOR LABOR

The small family norms and increasing rates of caesarean sections have made it mandatory that the health care providers must prepare the women much ahead she goes into Labor with the current changing trends in Labor. Preparation of Labor includes physical, psychological, and medical measures taken to ensure a smooth and safe labor process. It is extremely important that midwives/obstetricians prepare the women right from antenatal period so she is aware of all the details of delivery process, her rights where she can decide on her own regarding where she wants to deliver, with whom she wants to deliver and how she wants to deliver. She has to be groomed for *Normal Delivery*. She has to be prepared not only physically but also mentally/emotionally to allay her anxiety

The preparation of women includes the following strategies:

BPCR	Antenatal advices specially on diet and exercises	Making her aware of rights of, benefits of natural birth and how to prepare her for normal delivery
Showing her all props for alternative birthing positions and asking her to use them and explaining her all the positions and chosing her birth companion of her choice		Making her aware of Nonpharmacological methods of pain relief
Explaining her on all the complications of pregnancy, when and where she will report in emergency, whom she will contact and what all she will bring with her		
Information of all government programs for cashless deliveries		
Transportation details of government program		Helpline Nos
Mother and newborn kit of needs	Involvement of partner and family	Contraception advise

TAKE-HOME MESSAGE

- There are changing trends in labor management and updates are mandatory to know so as the capacity building and skills of the providers are enhanced
- LDR is the main concept, establishing MLCUs and OLCUs in close proximity for providing quality labor care to women
- Midwifery is a cadre to handle low risk cases and midwifery concept certainly shows multiple benefits in terms of compassionate care , promotes natural births with nonmedicalized pain relief, using props for delivering in upright positions or alternative birthing positions
- Counternutation and nutation help in normal deliveries
- One has to abolish the practices like enema, shaving, regular episiotomies, unnecessary medications and learn clipping, ambulation, supportive therapies, digital partography , delivering baby with no touch technique, placing baby on mothers abdomen, delayed cord clamping and fourth stage monitoring, etc.
- Antenatal preparation for labor and also in the first stage helps women to have great birthing experience
- Birth preparedness and complication readiness is the crux of have wonderful labor and labor experience.

SUGGESTED READING

1. Bai J, Lu Y, Liu H, et al. Editorial: New technologies improve maternal and newborn safety. Front Med Technol. 2024;6.

2. Guidelines on Standarduzation of labour rooms at delivery points. Ministry of Health and Family Welfare: Government of India; 2016.
3. Maternal Health Division: MOHFW. (2013). Maternal and Newborn Tool Kit. [online] Available from https://nhsrcindia.org/sites/default/files/2021-06/6.MNH%20Toolkit%20Nov%202013.pdf [Last accessed January, 2026].
4. Maternity Worldwide. Advocacy. [online] Available from https://www.maternityworldwide.org [Last accessed January, 2026].

2 CHAPTER

Analgesia in Labor

Bharti Wadhwa

INTRODUCTION

An important component of respectful maternity care, analgesia in labor reduces the physiological stress response with lower maternal exhaustion, better maternal cardiovascular stability and improved oxygenation to the fetus. Additionally, a positive birthing experience may help mitigate the long-term risk of postpartum depression and PTSD.

PAIN OF LABOR

First stage: (T10-L1 dermatomes): The pain of first stage of labor is visceral, diffuse, poorly localized over lower back and abdomen, similar to strong menstrual cramps and results from uterine stretching, distortion, ischemia and cervical dilatation

Second stage (S2, 3, 4 dermatomes): The pain of second stage of labor is sharp, localized pain, over lower back, perineum and inner side of thigh initially but mostly over perineum later and is due to stretching of pain sensitive perineum.

NEED FOR LABOR ANALGESIA

The pain induced increase in maternal catecholamines, heart rate and blood pressure, can reduce uteroplacental blood flow, and may aggravate conditions such as preeclampsia, cardiac disease and respiratory compromise. Hyperventilation due to pain and anxiety can cause respiratory alkalosis with reduced uteroplacental blood flow. Adequate pain relief improves maternal comfort, reduces anxiety, facilitates cooperation in labor and can indirectly improve fetomaternal wellbeing by providing cardiovascular stability and improved oxygenation to the fetus.

Recently, a 35% reduction in severe maternal mortality was reported in parturient who received epidural labor analgesia especially in women with preterm births and those who received epidural for medical indications.

Globally, contemporary guidelines such as WHO intrapartum care recommendations and NICE guidelines emphasize that effective pain relief is an integral part of a positive childbirth experience and that maternal request is a sufficient reason to provide analgesia.

INDICATIONS AND PATIENT SELECTION FOR LABOR ANALGESIA

Modern practice recognizes that maternal request alone is a sufficient indication for labor analgesia, provided there are no contraindications. Other specific indications include:

- High maternal anxiety, low pain threshold or previous traumatic birth experience
- Medical conditions in which pain induced tachycardia or hypertension can be harmful, for example significant cardiac disease, severe preeclampsia, certain valvular lesions, some congenital heart diseases
- Maternal respiratory compromise where excessive work of breathing should be avoided
- High risk pregnancies where stable hemodynamics and good cooperation are required, such as multiple pregnancy, preterm labor, intrauterine growth restriction and certain endocrine or neurological disorders
- Trial of labor after previous caesarean section, where good analgesia facilitates careful monitoring and timely decision making
- Anticipated operative vaginal delivery or instrumental procedures in the second stage

PREPARING FOR LABOR ANALGESIA

Sensitization for labor analgesia should begin in the antenatal period and early involvement of anesthesiologist is advised. Routine pre anesthesia check up with informed consent is mandatory. Preoperative advice includes acid aspiration prophylaxis every 12 hours for the duration of labor. In uncomplicated laboring patients: modest amounts of clear liquids can be allowed, while in high risk parturient, additional restriction of fluids is advised. All resuscitation equipment and drugs should be kept ready and the parturient should have a functioning IV access.

METHODS FOR RELIEF OF LABOR PAIN

Labor analgesia can be divided into nonpharmacological methods, systemic pharmacological methods and regional (neuraxial and nerve block) techniques. Choice depends on maternal preference, stage of labor, contraindications, and available resources.

Nonpharmacological Methods

These are mostly effective in first stage of labor but particularly important in resource limited settings. Systematic reviews suggest modest reduction in pain, increased maternal satisfaction and are often used as adjunct or part of a multimodal strategy. These include:

- Continuous labor support by a doula or birth companion

- Childbirth education, breathing and relaxation exercises, guided imagery
- Position changes, ambulation, use of birthing ball
- Massage, acupressure, warm baths or showers, application of heat or cold
- Transcutaneous electrical nerve stimulation devices
- Water immersion where facilities exist
- Sterile water injections

Sterile water injections provide significant relief of lower back pain during first stage labor with no maternal-fetal adverse effect apart from the administration pain. The technique involves intradermal injections of 0.1 mL sterile water over posterior superior iliac spines (both sides) and 1 cm medial and 2–3 cm inferior to the first injections (on both sides). The injection is transiently painful for 30 sec followed by pain relief within 2 min that lasts till 45–120 minutes. Administration of SWIs is an easy, low-cost technique with a short learning curve. There is no restriction of mobility and can repeated as often as desired which makes it a suitable option for the overworked, low resource labor rooms and also for women who wish to avoid epidural analgesia.

Systemic Pharmacological Methods

1. *Intramuscular or intravenous opioids:* Commonly used agents include pethidine, tramadol, fentanyl and more recently remifentanil. They are easy to administer, relatively inexpensive and widely available. However, they provide only moderate pain relief and may cause maternal nausea, vomiting, sedation and transient fetal respiratory or neurobehavioral depression, especially if given close to delivery.
2. *Intravenous remifentanil patient-controlled analgesia infusion:* This offers better analgesia than traditional opioids and has the advantage of rapid termination of action due to esterase-based metabolism. It is recommended in women who cannot or do not wish to have neuraxial analgesia, provided close monitoring and appropriate facilities are available.
3. *Inhalational nitrous oxide and oxygen*: A 50:50 mixture (Entonox or equivalent) is self-administered via a demand valve face mask. It is simple, rapidly acting and has minimal accumulation, though analgesic potency is modest and effective scavenging systems are important.

REGIONAL TECHNIQUES

1. *Epidural analgesia:* Includes continuous lumbar epidural, combined spinal epidural (CSE) and Dural puncture epidural techniques.
2. *Single shot spinal (intrathecal) analgesia:* A small dose of opioid with or without low dose local anesthetic can provide rapid onset analgesia of limited duration, useful in advanced labor or where epidural is not feasible.

3. Pudendal nerve block for perineal analgesia in the late second stage or for instrumental delivery
4. Paracervical block, now rarely used because of risk of fetal bradycardia, primarily for early first stage pain

EPIDURAL LABOR ANALGESIA

Lumbar epidural analgesia using dilute local anesthetic with opioid is widely regarded as the gold standard for labor analgesia because it provides superior pain relief with minimal motor block and ability to ambulate when modern low dose low concentration local anesthetics regimens are used. Additionally, there is flexibility of extension of the block for surgical anesthesia. Common drug regimens include low concentration local anesthetic, often combined with opioids such as bupivacaine 0.0625–0.125% or ropivacaine 0.1–0.2%, combined with fentanyl 2 μg/mL.

EFFECT OF LABOR ANALGESIA ON PROGRESS OF LABOR AND MODE OF DELIVERY

Historically, epidural labor analgesia was associated with prolonged labor, higher rates of instrumental vaginal delivery and caesarean section. Many of these associations came from older studies that used higher concentrations of local anesthetic, which produced dense motor block. Contemporary evidence using low concentration local anesthetic opioid mixtures paints a more nuanced picture.

Several large observational studies and randomized trials show that epidural analgesia may modestly prolong the first and second stages of labor, particularly in nulliparous women, but without major clinical consequence when labor is well managed. A recent study found an approximately one hour longer active phase and a modest increase in second stage duration among women with epidurals. Withholding analgesia until the patient has achieved an arbitrary cervical dilatation during the first stage of labor is unnecessary. Best time to administer ELA: linked to parturient demand not cervical dilatation provided established labor is ensured.

Systematic reviews indicate that neuraxial analgesia does not increase the incidence of caesarean delivery. The effect on instrumental vaginal delivery is more complex. Some earlier meta-analyses suggested a small increase in forceps or vacuum delivery, whereas more recent work with low dose protocols and flexible pushing policies shows little or no difference. Instrumental delivery appears to be influenced by multiple factors, including obstetric practice, fetal position and use of oxytocin, rather than epidural alone.

In summary, with contemporary low dose neuraxial techniques, epidural labor analgesia does not increase caesarean section rates and has at most a modest effect on labor duration and instrumental delivery rates, particularly when coupled with good obstetric management.

MONITORING DURING EPIDURAL LABOR ANALGESIA

- Measure BP and HR every 3–5 minutes for first 15 minutes, then every 15 minutes during the infusion and until the block wears off.
- Uterine contractions, FHR, cervical dilatation
- Patient should turn from side to side every 30 minutes to avoid a one-sided block
- Temperature 4 hourly—If increased then hourly
- *Sensory level:* sensation to cold: Every 1 hour
- Adequacy of analgesia → Pain Score: Every 1 hour
- *Motor block:* Ability of the patient to lift legs Every 1 hour
- Sit patient forward and check integrity of epidural dressing/dislodgement of epidural catheter intermittently every 2–3 hours
- CTG for at least 30 minutes with establishment of regional analgesia and after administration of each further bolus of 10 mL or more.

AMBULATORY LABOR ANALGESIA

Any neuraxial analgesic technique with minimal motor block that allows safe ambulation. First coined to describe low-dose CSE opioid analgesia because motor function was maintained and ability to walk was not impaired. Equally effective with low dose epidurals.

Benefits of ambulation: Include better analgesia, stronger uterine contractions, minimal aortocaval compression, ability to void spontaneously, lower incidence of DVT, improved maternal satisfaction, lower instrumental delivery rate. For the Labor room personnel, the improved patient mobility reduces the manpower requirements.

MANAGING THE SECOND STAGE OF LABOR

Early pushing can result in maternal exhaustion and frequent variable decelerations. Thus, parturient should be actively encouraged to push during contractions (Delayed pushing) rather than early pushing with full dilatation as it increases likelihood of spontaneous vaginal delivery. Routine use of oxytocin and arbitrary termination of the second stage of labor for women with regional analgesia is discouraged.

COMPLICATIONS AND SIDE EFFECTS OF EPIDURAL LABOR ANALGESIA

Maternal Complications

Adverse effects common to epidural block:

- Hypotension from sympathetic block
- Pruritus, nausea and urinary retention, particularly with opioid containing solutions

- Shivering and mild sedation
- Post dural puncture headache

Adverse effects specific to labor analgesia:

- *Epidural related maternal fever:* Women who receive ELA are more likely to develop hyperthermia [incidence: 15–25%] with an average temperature increase of approximately 1°C over 7 hours. The duration and type of epidural technique does not influence the risk of developing maternal fever and the cause is likely inflammatory rather than infectious, but the presence of maternal fever often triggers neonatal sepsis evaluations
- *Backache:* There is no convincing evidence that epidural labor analgesia causes chronic back pain; large studies have shown similar rates of long-term back pain in women with and without epidurals.

Fetal Effects

When maternal blood pressure is maintained and drug doses are appropriate, epidural labor analgesia has minimal direct effect on the fetus. Potential issues include transient fetal heart rate abnormalities secondary to maternal hypotension or rapid changes in uterine tone, which improve with maternal resuscitative measures.

CONCLUSION

Pain relief in labor is both a clinical necessity and part of respectful motherhood. While a range of options exists, neuraxial techniques, particularly lumbar epidural analgesia with low concentration local anesthetic opioid mixtures, remain the gold standard, offering excellent analgesia with minimal impact on labor outcomes and a favorable safety profile for mother and baby. Epidural analgesia can further aid in reducing severe maternal mortality and expanding epidural access could improve maternal health. Use of sterile water block is a suitable option for the Indian labor rooms and can provide safe and effective analgesia with minimal cost and manpower requirements.

SUGGESTED READING

1. ACOG Committee Opinion No. 766: approaches to limit intervention during labor and birth. Obstet Gynecol. 2019;133(2):e164-e173.
2. Ayres-de-Campos D, Spong CY, Chandraharan E; FIGO Intrapartum Fetal Monitoring Expert Consensus Panel. FIGO consensus guidelines on intrapartum fetal monitoring: Cardiotocography. Int J Gynaecol Obstet. 2015;131(1):13-24.
3. Beyable AA, Bayable SD, Ashebir YG. Pharmacologic and non-pharmacologic labor pain management techniques in a resource-limited setting: A systematic review. Ann Med Surg (Lond). 2022;74:103312.

4. Blackburn R, Mehmeti A, Russell S, et al. Intrapartum Care: Updated Summary of NICE Guidance. Obstet Anesth Digest. 2024;44(4):184.
5. Cavusoglu Colak G, Arkan K, Bagli I, et al. The Impact of Epidural Analgesia on the Dynamics of Labor and Perinatal Outcomes in Nulliparous Women: A Prospective Cohort Study. Medicina. 2025;61(12):2109.
6. Halliday L, Nelson SM, Kearns RJ. Epidural analgesia in labor: A narrative review. Int J Gynecol Obstet. 2022;159:356-64.
7. Hasegawa J, Farina A, Turchi G, et al. Effects of epidural analgesia on labor length, instrumental delivery, and neonatal short-term outcome. J Anesth. 2013;27:43-7.
8. Kearns RJ, Kyzayeva A, Halliday LOE, et al. Epidural analgesia during labor and severe maternal morbidity: population-based study. BMJ. 2024;385:e077190.
9. Leighton BL, Halpern SH. Epidural analgesia: effects on labor progress and maternal and neonatal outcome. Semin Perinatol. 2002;26(2):122-35.
10. Mamuk R, Şahin NH. Effect of Intradermal Sterile Water Injection on Labor Experiences: A Randomized Controlled Study. Clin Exp Obstet Gynecol. 2023;50(3):65.
11. Nori W, Kassim MAK, Helmi ZR, et al. Non-Pharmacological Pain Management in Labor: A Systematic Review. J Clin Med. 2023;12(23):7203.
12. Roberts CL, Torvaldsen S, Cameron CA, et al. Delayed versus early pushing in women with epidural analgesia: a systematic review and meta-analysis. BJOG. 2004;111:1333-40.
13. Zuarez-Easton S, Erez O, Zafran N, et al. Pharmacologic and nonpharmacologic options for pain relief during labor: an expert review Am J Obstet Gynecol. 2023;228(5S):S1246-59.

3 CHAPTER

Dynamic Consent in Birthing and Understanding the WHO Labor Care Guide for Safe Childbirth: Advancing Respectful, Person-centered Maternity Care

Jayasree Sundar

INTRODUCTION

Childbirth is a landmark life event that holds significant physical, psychological, and social implications for women and families. Labor and childbirth remain critical determinants of maternal and perinatal outcomes. Despite advances in obstetric care, significant differences continue to remain in the practice of labor monitoring, timely recognition of complications, and the use or overuse of interventions. Over the past decade, maternal health research and global clinical guidelines have shifted toward a more woman-centered, evidence-based, and respectful model of intrapartum care. In 2018, WHO released comprehensive recommendations on intrapartum care for a positive childbirth experience, emphasizing individualized labor support, avoidance of unnecessary interventions, and the importance of respectful maternity care (RMC). Central to RMC is the protection of women's autonomy and the enhancement of communication between women and healthcare providers. Dynamic consent has emerged as an important ethical model for guiding interactions during labor and birth. Simultaneously, the WHO Labor Care Guide (LCG) was introduced as a replacement for the traditional partograph, intending to improve both clinical quality and women's experience during labor. Understanding these two frameworks is essential for clinicians, policymakers, and researchers committed to advancing safe and respectful childbirth practices.

This chapter summarizes the key features, structure, and clinical implications of the WHO Labor Care Guide, with particular attention to how its use can enhance obstetric practice.

DYNAMIC CONSENT IN BIRTHING

Conceptualization and Definition

Dynamic consent is an adaptive, continuous, and participatory approach to decision-making during childbirth. Unlike static or one-time consent processes—often obtained at admission or early in pregnancy—dynamic consent recognizes that labor is inherently unpredictable and that a woman's preferences, comfort, and clinical circumstances may evolve rapidly. It is built on ongoing dialogue and shared understanding, in which the woman remains an active participant in decisions about her body and her care throughout the entire intrapartum period.

Principles Underpinning Dynamic Consent

Dynamic consent rests on several ethical, clinical, and relational principles:

1. *Continuity of Communication:* Because labor progresses in stages and interventions arise at different times, communication must be iterative rather than episodic. Healthcare providers are expected to revisit discussions before any procedure, verify understanding, and allow reassessment of decisions.
2. *Informed Choice and Transparency:* Information provided to the woman must be timely, balanced, and comprehensible. This includes discussing risks, benefits, alternatives, and the possibility of refusal without punitive consequences.
3. *Respect for Autonomy and Bodily Integrity:* Women retain full control over their bodies throughout labor. Consent cannot be presumed from silence, routine practice, or institutional norms; it must be actively obtained.
4. *Supportive and Empowering Environment:* Emotional, psychological, and physical support—including the presence of a chosen birth companion—enhances a woman's capacity to engage in informed decision-making.
5. *Documentation and Accountability:* Clinicians must record consent discussions and decisions, promoting transparency and safeguarding women's rights.

Practical Applications in Labor

Dynamic consent is relevant to a wide range of intrapartum procedures and decisions, such as:

- Vaginal examinations
- Induction or augmentation of labor
- Artificial rupture of membranes
- Pain management options (pharmacological and non-pharmacological)
- Continuous or intermittent fetal monitoring
- Positioning and mobility during labor
- Assisted vaginal birth
- Caesarean section
- Episiotomy
- Newborn care (e.g., cord clamping, skin-to-skin contact)

Each of these moments presents an opportunity for shared decision-making, acknowledging that a woman's needs, preferences, and interpretations of risk may shift over time.

Benefits of Dynamic Consent

Adopting dynamic consent contributes to:

- *Enhanced trust* between women and healthcare providers
- *Reduced fear and psychological trauma,* particularly post-birth trauma linked to loss of control
- *Improved maternal satisfaction and sense of empowerment*
- *Decreased risk of obstetric violence,* coercion, and unnecessary interventions
- *Strengthened medicolegal protection* for both clients and clinicians through accountability

Overall, dynamic consent promotes a relational model of care that values communication as much as clinical competence.

UNDERSTANDING THE WHO LABOR CARE GUIDE

Purpose and Evolution

The WHO Labor Care Guide (LCG), a next-generation clinical tool, was introduced as an update to the conventional WHO partograph. The new LCG addresses the limitations of conventional WHO partograph through a more holistic, woman-centered, and evidence-based framework for labor monitoring. It encourages continuous assessment not only of labor progress and fetal well-being but also of supportive care, shared decision-making, maternal experience, and evidence-based interventions. It is designed to facilitate *clinical decision-making, timely action, and positive childbirth experiences,* while actively discouraging unnecessary or harmful practices.

Objectives of the WHO Labor Care Guide

The LCG aims to:

- Improve quality and safety of intrapartum care
- Encourage individualized assessment rather than fixed labor progression expectations
- Integrate respectful and supportive care throughout labor
- Early identification of problems and timely, appropriate and proportionate clinical intervention
- Strengthen shared decision-making
- Enhance outcomes for mothers and newborns
- *Reduce unnecessary interventions* and promote physiologic labor where possible

The LCG integrates additional domains of care—supportive care, maternal well-being, fetal assessment, shared decision-making; thus acknowledging that labor is not solely a mechanical process but a complex biopsychosocial experience replacing the focus only on cervical dilatation.

Who Should Use the Labor Care Guide?

The LCG is *primarily designed for healthy, low-risk pregnancies,* while still allowing flexibility for high-risk cases, where additional monitoring and documentation may be required. The tool is designed for use across all levels of health care facilities, namely primary, secondary, and tertiary. The specific clinical actions available in a particular facility will vary by the level of care.

When to Initiate the Labor Care Guide?

The LCG should be initiated at the *onset of the active phase of labor,* defined as cervical dilatation of *5 cm or more,* regardless of parity, and membrane status. This aligns with updated WHO labor definitions avoids premature interventions during latent labor while support is continuously given. Once initiated, the LCG is used *continuously throughout the first and second stages* of active labor.

Structure and Components of the LCG

The LCG is composed of *seven sections,* each capturing essential aspects of labor monitoring and decision-making. Each section includes a *vertical axis* with reference thresholds - "alert" criteria - and a *horizontal time axis* for entry of observations.

Section 1: Identifying Information and Admission Characteristics

This section records essential baseline information, including:

- Parity
- Mode of labor onset (spontaneous/induced/augmented)
- Time of diagnosis of active labor
- Time of membrane rupture
- Any maternal or fetal risk factors

These details provide clinical context and inform subsequent decisions.

Section 2: Supportive Care

A hallmark of the LCG is the integration of *respectful maternity care (RMC) into routine intrapartum care.* This section ensures documentation and consistent provision of supportive care practices, such as:

- Allowing a labor companion
- Access to nonpharmacological and pharmacological pain relief
- Mobility and position changes
- Encouragement of oral intake
- Comfort measures (e.g., reassurance, touch, relaxation techniques)

These interventions improve maternal satisfaction and may reduce the need for medical interventions.

Section 3: Care of the Baby

Fetal well-being is monitored by:

- Baseline fetal heart rate
- Presence and type of decelerations
- Amniotic fluid characteristics
- Fetal position
- Molding and caput

Clear thresholds guide clinicians on when to reflect, reassess, and act.

Section 4: Care of the Woman

This section focuses on maternal health through periodic observation of:

- Pulse
- Blood pressure
- Temperature
- Urine output and characteristics

These parameters allow early detection of maternal compromise, infection, dehydration, and hypertensive disorders.

Section 5: Labor Progress

In contrast to the traditional partograph's fixed "alert" and "action" lines, the LCG adopts more flexible, physiologically aligned thresholds. Labor progress is assessed through:

- Frequency and duration of contractions
- Cervical dilatation
- Fetal head descent

The use of evidence-based expected ranges rather than rigid linear expectations respects individual variability.

Section 6: Medication

This section captures:

- Use and dosing of oxytocin
- Other medications given during labor
- IV fluids administered

This promotes safe, judicious use of oxytocin and ensures accurate documentation of all treatments.

Section 7: Shared Decision-making

The LCG recognizes that *effective communication* is integral to quality care. This section documents:

- Counseling provided
- Discussions with the labor companion
- Agreed plans of care
- Any decisions to intervene and their rationale

This supports transparency, patient autonomy, and trust.

The Monitoring-to-action Cycle

A distinctive contribution of the LCG is the Assess → Record → Check → Plan loop:

1. *Assess* the woman, fetus, and labor progress.
2. *Record* findings against the structured time axis.
3. *Check* values against reference thresholds.
4. *Plan* appropriate actions—including non-intervention, supportive measures, or medical management.

Table 1 enlists the differences between the traditional partogram and the WHO LCG.

Innovations Compared to the Partograph

Key innovations include:

- A shift from rigid time-based expectations to *individualized labor patterns*
- Explicit inclusion of *emotional and supportive care indicators*
- Greater emphasis on *clinical reasoning* rather than routine interventions
- Integrated *decision-making,* reflecting best practices in patient-centered care

Checklist for Labor Ward Use of the LCG

Before Starting (Latent Phase):

1. Confirm maternal identity and risk factors
2. Ensure supportive care: companion, fluids, mobility
3. Offer pain relief options
4. Assess maternal vitals and FHR

TABLE 1: Comparison: WHO Labor Care Guide versus Traditional Partograph.

Feature	*WHO Labor Care Guide (LCG)*	*Traditional Partograph*
Primary philosophy	Woman-centered, holistic monitoring	Biomedical, progress-focused
Start point	Active labor at 5 cm	3–4 cm dilatation
Focus areas	Supportive care, maternal status, fetal health, labor progress	Cervical dilatation, contractions
Labor thresholds	Flexible, evidence-based	Fixed alert/action lines
Shared decision-making	Explicit documentation	Not included
RMC	Dedicated section	Not addressed
Fetal monitoring	FHR + decels + amniotic fluid	FHR only
Maternal monitoring	Pulse/BP/temperature/urine	Limited
Intervention Documentation	Oxytocin dose/timing	Minimal
Overall goal	Positive childbirth + safety	Detect slow labor

At 5 cm (Start of LCG):

1. Record admission characteristics
2. Document membrane status
3. Begin supportive care documentation
4. Assess fetal position, molding, caput
5. Establish cervical dilatation baseline

Active Labor:

1. Maternal vitals every 30–60 minutes
2. FHR as recommended
3. Contractions every 30 min
4. Cervical exam every 4 hours
5. Review medications (oxytocin, others)
6. Document decisions and discussions

Second Stage:

1. Continuous FHR
2. Support physiologic pushing
3. Document descent and fetal condition

Post-Birth Audit:

1. Review all sections for completeness
2. Document deviations and actions

INTERSECTION OF DYNAMIC CONSENT AND THE WHO LABOR CARE GUIDE

Dynamic consent is embedded within the conceptual foundation and practical use of the LCG. For example, the LCG's first section on supportive care ensures that clinicians assess a woman's comfort and preferences continuously. Similarly, the final section on shared decision-making requires clinicians to document counselling discussions and the woman's choices.

The LCG therefore operationalizes dynamic consent by converting ethical principles into documented clinical practice. It reinforces the idea that labor care should not merely be a series of clinical assessments, but a holistic process respecting woman's rights, fosters autonomy, and supports individualized care. Through this integration, the LCG and dynamic consent jointly promote the transformation of maternity care into a model that balances safety with dignity.

CONCLUSION

Dynamic consent and the WHO Labor Care Guide together represent a pivotal shift toward compassionate, evidence-based, and rights-respecting childbirth care. Both frameworks underscore that childbirth is not only a clinical event but also a deeply personal experience requiring respectful engagement and shared decision-making. As worldwide we strive to improve maternal outcomes and eliminate mistreatment in maternity care, the integration of Guide and dynamic consenting offers a robust path toward achieving high-quality, woman-centered intrapartum care. Its adoption can strengthen health systems, standardize safe practices, ensuring that every woman is supported, respected, and cared for during one of the most important event of her life.

SUGGESTED READING

1. Bohren MA, Tunçalp Ö, Miller S. Transforming intrapartum care: respectful maternity care. Best Pract Res Clin Obstet Gynecol. 2020;67:113-26.
2. Bohren MA, Vogel JP, Hunter EC, et al. The mistreatment of women during childbirth in health facilities globally: a mixed-methods systematic review. PLoS Med. 2015;12(6):e1001847.
3. FIGO Working Group on Best Practice in Maternal-Fetal Medicine. FIGO guidelines on respectful maternity care. Int J Gynecol Obstet. 2019;145(1):3-6.
4. Montgomery J. Autonomy, consent and the limits of medical paternalism. J Med Ethics. 2017;43(8):497-500.
5. Oladapo OT, et al. Development of the WHO Labor Care Guide. BJOG. 2020.
6. World Health Organization. Improving the quality of care for mothers and newborns in health facilities. Geneva: World Health Organization; 2016.
7. World Health Organization. WHO Labor Care Guide: user's manual. Geneva: World Health Organization; 2020.
8. World Health Organization. WHO recommendations: intrapartum care for a positive childbirth experience. Geneva: World Health Organization; 2018.

4 CHAPTER

Shoulder Dystocia: Recognition and Stepwise Management

Kanchan Sharma

INTRODUCTION

Shoulder dystocia is a rare but serious obstetric emergency characterized by failure of the fetal shoulders to deliver after the fetal head has emerged, despite gentle traction in the absence of impaction of the fetal head.

It is unpredictable in many cases and is associated with significant maternal and neonatal morbidity and occasional mortality.

Prompt recognition and a calm, systematic response are critical for good outcomes.

DEFINITION

Shoulder dystocia is classically defined as:

- Vaginal cephalic delivery in which additional obstetric maneuvers are required to deliver the shoulders after gentle downward traction has failed.

Clinically, it is often recognized by:

- Failure of the shoulders to deliver with normal traction
- *"Turtle sign":* Retraction of the delivered head against the perineum.

INCIDENCE

- *Reported incidence:* 0.2–3% of all vaginal cephalic deliveries.
- Higher rates are seen in:
    - Macrosomic fetuses
    - Diabetic pregnancies
    - Instrumental (operative) vaginal deliveries.

Table 1 shows the risk factors.

RISK FACTORS

Although some factors increase risk, but up to half of cases occur without identifiable risk factors.

Antepartum Risk Factors

- Fetal macrosomia (>4.0–4.5 kg)
- Maternal diabetes mellitus (pre-gestational or gestational)

TABLE 1: Risk factors for shoulder dystocia.

Risk category	*Risk factor*
Maternal	• Diabetes mellitus (GDM or pregestational) • Obesity • Excessive gestational weight gain • Short stature
Fetal	• Macrosomia (>4.0–4.5 kg) • Male sex (slight increase)
Obstetric history	• Previous shoulder dystocia • Previous macrosomic baby
Intrapartum	• Prolonged second stage • Instrumental vaginal delivery • Induction/augmentation with oxytocin

(GDM: gestational diabetes mellitus)

- Maternal obesity
- Excessive gestational weight gain
- Prior history of shoulder dystocia

Intrapartum Risk Factors

- Prolonged second stage of labor
- Operative vaginal delivery (forceps, vacuum)
- Induction or augmentation with oxytocin
- Precipitous or very rapid second stage in a large baby

Important Clinical Point

History of shoulder dystocia in a previous pregnancy is the strongest single risk factor, with recurrence risk of approximately 10%. (Details are summarized in **Table 1**.)

PATHOPHYSIOLOGY AND CLINICAL FEATURES

In Normal Labor

The fetal shoulders enter the pelvis in the oblique diameter and rotate to allow the anterior shoulder to pass under the symphysis pubis.

In Shoulder Dystocia

- The anterior shoulder becomes impacted behind the symphysis pubis (most common), or
- The posterior shoulder is impacted on the sacral promontory.

Consequences

- Compression of the umbilical cord → reduced oxygen delivery
- Compression of fetal chest → impaired breathing movements
- Potential for hypoxic brain injury if delivery is delayed.

Clinical Clues during Birth

- Difficulty delivering the face and chin
- Failure of restitution and external rotation of the head
- Head tightly applied to vulva ("turtle sign")
- Failure of shoulders to deliver with gentle traction.

PREDICTION AND PREVENTION

- No single factor reliably predicts shoulder dystocia.
- Ultrasound-estimated fetal weight (EFW) has limited accuracy and should not be the only basis for intervention.

Elective cesarean section may be considered in:

- Diabetic mother with EFW ≥ 4.5 kg
- Non-diabetic mother with EFW ≥ 5.0 kg
- Strong history of severe shoulder dystocia with neonatal injury in previous pregnancy.

GENERAL PREVENTIVE STRATEGIES

- Optimal glycemic control in diabetic pregnancies
- Monitoring and counseling regarding excessive gestational weight gain
- Judicious use of oxytocin and instrumental delivery
- Regular team training and drills on shoulder dystocia management.

INTRAPARTUM RECOGNITION AND INITIAL RESPONSE

Once shoulder dystocia is suspected:

DO immediately:

- Announce "shoulder dystocia" clearly.
- Call for help (obstetrician, anesthetist, neonatologist, senior midwife).
- Ask the woman to stop pushing temporarily.
- Maintain the head in a neutral position, avoid excessive traction.

Do not:

Apply fundal pressure (increases impaction and risk of uterine rupture and fetal trauma).

Algorithmic approach is recommended **(Flowchart 1)**.

Flowchart 1: Algorithm for management of shoulder dystocia.

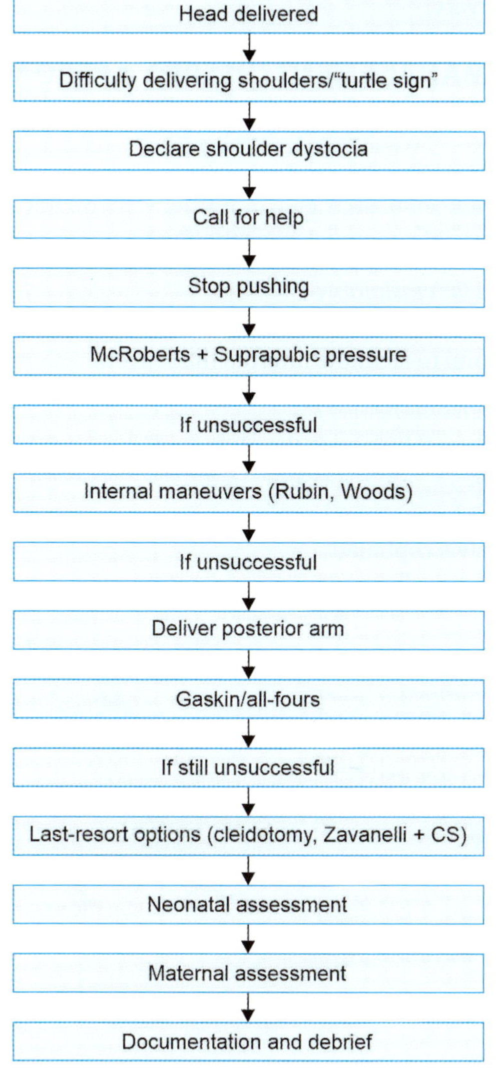

PRINCIPLES OF MANAGEMENT

Overall Goals

- Relieve impaction of the shoulder
- Deliver the baby as quickly as possible, ideally within 5 minutes of head delivery
- Minimize maternal and neonatal trauma.

Key Principles

- Use sequential, evidence-based maneuvers rather than random attempts.
- Maintain clear communication among team members.

- Document time of head delivery, maneuvers performed, and time of complete delivery.

STEPWISE MANAGEMENT (HELPER APPROACH)

Adapted from commonly used obstetric emergency algorithms.

H—Help

- Call for experienced obstetrician, anesthetist, neonatal team.
- Prepare for possible neonatal resuscitation.

E—Evaluate need for episiotomy

- Episiotomy does not relieve the bony obstruction.
- It may be helpful to facilitate internal maneuvers.

L—Legs (McRoberts maneuver)

- Hyperflex maternal hips onto the abdomen.
- This:
    - Straightens lumbosacral angle
    - Rotates pelvis cephalad

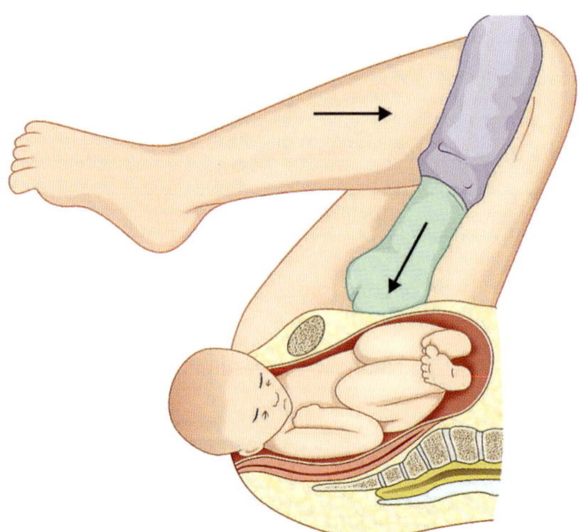

- Increases anteroposterior diameter of pelvic outlet.
- Often combined with suprapubic pressure.

P—Suprapubic pressure

- Apply firm, continuous or rocking pressure just above the pubic bone, directed posteriorly and laterally towards the fetal back.
- *Aim:* dislodge the anterior shoulder and rotate it into an oblique diameter.
- Must never be replaced by fundal pressure.

E—Enter maneuvers (internal rotational maneuvers)

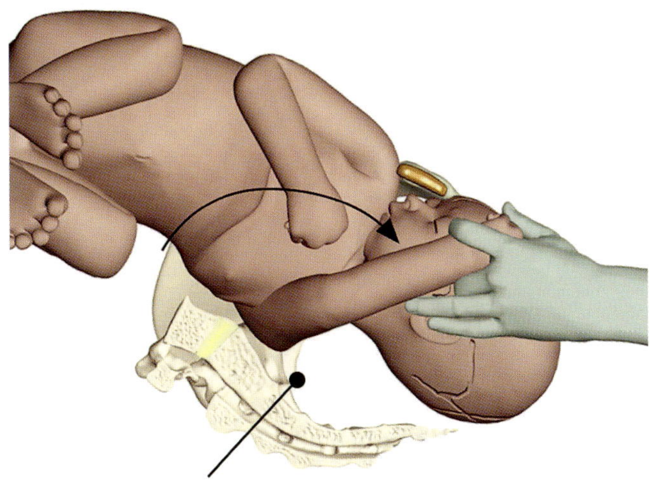

1. Rubin maneuver
   - Insert fingers behind the anterior shoulder.
   - Apply pressure towards the fetal chest to adduct the shoulder and reduce the bisacromial diameter.

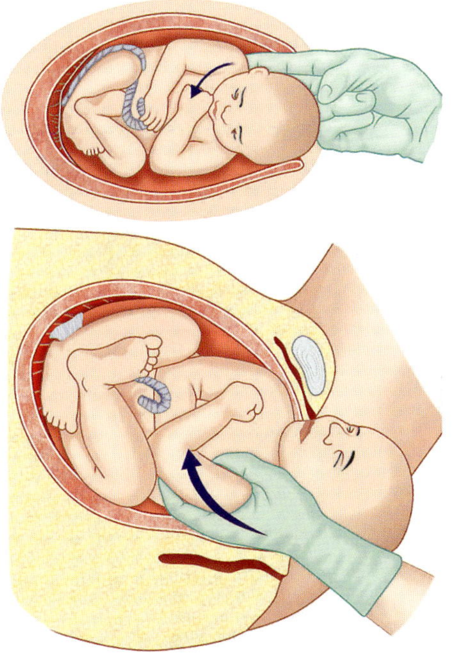

2. Woods corkscrew maneuver

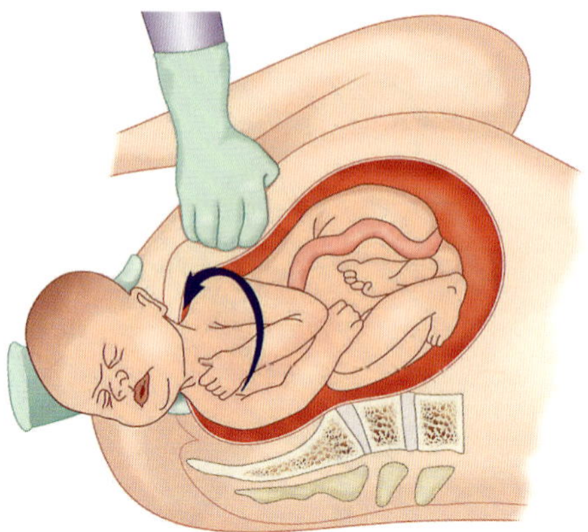

- One hand applies pressure behind the posterior shoulder to rotate the fetus in a "corkscrew" fashion.
- Often used in combination with Rubin maneuver.

R—Remove posterior arm

- Insert hand into the sacral hollow, locate the posterior arm.
- Flex elbow and sweep the forearm across the chest and out of the vagina.
- Reduces the shoulder-to-shoulder diameter and often allows delivery.

R—Roll the patient (Gaskin maneuver)

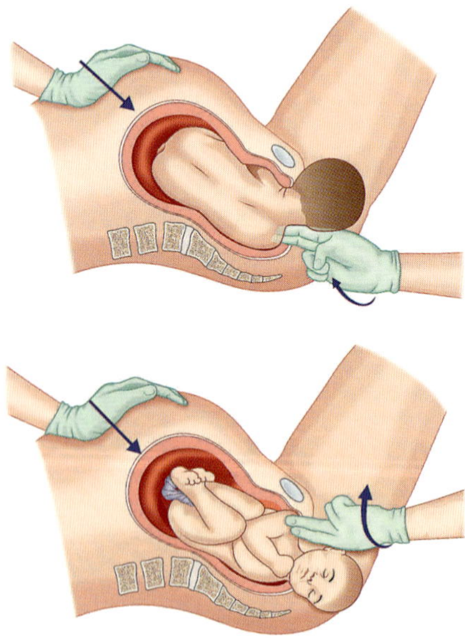

- Ask the woman to move to the all-fours position (on hands and knees).
- This may increase pelvic diameters and help free the shoulders.

If all above fail (rare):

- Consider last-resort procedures:
- Cleidotomy (intentional fracture of fetal clavicle)
- Symphysiotomy (rare, specialized setting)
- Zavanelli maneuver (cephalic replacement and emergency caesarean section).

Sequence is summarized in **Table 2 and Flowchart 1**.

MATERNAL COMPLICATIONS

- Postpartum hemorrhage (PPH) due to uterine atony or trauma
- Perineal trauma: third- or fourth-degree perineal tears
- Cervical, vaginal, or uterine lacerations
- Uterine rupture (rare, usually with fundal pressure or mismanaged cases)
- Psychological trauma, anxiety in subsequent pregnancies.

FETAL AND NEONATAL COMPLICATIONS

- Brachial plexus injury (BPI)
- Erb's palsy (C5–C6) most common
- May be temporary neuropraxia or permanent damage.
- Clavicular and humeral fractures
- Hypoxic-ischemic encephalopathy (HIE)
- Low Apgar scores and need for resuscitation
- In extreme cases, neonatal death.

Most brachial plexus injuries resolve spontaneously within weeks to months, but a subset may result in permanent functional impairment.

DOCUMENTATION, AUDIT, AND COUNSELING

Documentation should include:

- Time of head delivery and time of complete delivery
- Personnel present and time help arrived

TABLE 2: Stepwise management of shoulder dystocia (HELPERR).

Step	*Maneuver/Action*	*Key points*
H	Help	Call senior obstetrician, anesthetist, peds
E	Evaluate need for episiotomy	Facilitates internal maneuvers
L	McRoberts maneuver	Hyperflex hips, increases pelvic outlet
P	Suprapubic pressure	Downward, lateral pressure, no fundal
E	Enter maneuvers (Rubin, Woods corkscrew)	Internal rotation of shoulders
R	Remove posterior arm	Reduces bisacromial diameter
R	Roll patient (Gaskin, all-fours)	Alters pelvic dimensions

(Peds: pediatric/neonatal team)

- All maneuvers performed and their sequence
- Use of McRoberts, suprapubic pressure, internal maneuvers, episiotomy, etc.
- Condition of the baby at birth (Apgar scores, resuscitation measures)
- Maternal and neonatal injuries identified.

POSTEVENT DEBRIEFING

- With the clinical team—to review performance and reinforce learning.
- With the woman (and family)—to explain what happened, possible implications and plan for follow-up.

FUTURE PREGNANCY COUNSELING

Discuss recurrence risk (~10%) and options:

- Close monitoring of fetal growth
- Consideration of elective caesarean section in selected high-risk cases, especially with prior shoulder dystocia and neonatal injury.

CONCLUSION

Shoulder dystocia remains a challenging obstetric emergency because of its relative unpredictability and potential for severe neonatal and maternal morbidity. Preparedness, early recognition, adherence to a structured stepwise algorithm (such as HELPERR), and effective team communication can significantly improve outcomes. Regular skills training, simulation drills, careful documentation, and appropriate counseling are essential components of modern obstetric practice in managing shoulder dystocia.

TAKE-HOME MESSAGE

- Shoulder dystocia is an acute obstetric emergency with potential for serious neonatal and maternal complications.
- It is often unpredictable; risk factors help identify high-risk situations but cannot reliably exclude the condition.
- Early recognition using signs such as the turtle sign and prompt declaration of "shoulder dystocia" are crucial for activating the emergency response.
- Management must follow a structured, stepwise approach (McRoberts, suprapubic pressure, internal rotational maneuvers, delivery of posterior arm, all-fours position).
- Fundal pressure is contraindicated and increases the risk of trauma and uterine rupture.
- Brachial plexus injury, fractures, and hypoxic–ischemic encephalopathy are key neonatal concerns; postpartum hemorrhage and severe perineal trauma are major maternal risks.
- Accurate documentation, debriefing, and appropriate counseling for future pregnancies are integral parts of care.
- Regular drills and simulation training significantly improve team performance and outcomes in shoulder dystocia.

SUGGESTED READING

1. ACOG Practice Bulletin. Fetal Macrosomia. Obstet Gynecol. 2020;135(1):e18-e35.
2. American College of Obstetricians and Gynecologists. Practice Bulletin No. 178: Shoulder Dystocia. Obstet Gynecol. 2017;129(5):e123-e133.
3. Gherman RB, Chauhan S, Lewis DF. Shoulder dystocia: an evidence-based evaluation of the obstetric nightmare. Obstet Gynecol Surv. 2006;61(11):689-97.
4. Gurewitsch ED, Allen RH, Gurewitsch S, et al. Symphysiotomy for shoulder dystocia: a review. Obstet Gynecol Surv. 2004;59(6):433-8.
5. McRoberts WR, Hellman LM, Pritchard JA. A simple approach to the management of shoulder dystocia. Am J Obstet Gynecol. 1957;73(4):859-67.
6. Ouzounian JG, Korst LM, Phelan JP. Permanent brachial plexus injury: relationship to birth weight and maternal diabetes. Am J Obstet Gynecol. 1998;179(3 Pt 1):713-7.
7. RCOG. (2012). RCOG Green-top Guideline No. 42. Shoulder Dystocia. [online] Available from https://www.rcog.org.uk/guidance/browse-all-guidance/green-top-guidelines/shoulder-dystocia-green-top-guideline-no-42/ [Last accessed January, 2026].
8. Spong CY, Beall M, Rodrigues D, et al. An objective definition of shoulder dystocia: prolonged head-to-body delivery intervals and/or use of ancillary obstetric maneuvers. Obstet Gynecol. 1997;89(5 Pt 1):671-5.
9. Woods CE. A new maneuver for the relief of arm lock in shoulder dystocia. Am J Obstet Gynecol. 1943;46:796-804.

5 CHAPTER

Cardiotocography Interpretation and Intrapartum Fetal Monitoring

Ajith S

INTRODUCTION

The CTG was introduced into clinical practice in the late 1950s with the hope of reducing perinatal morbidity and mortality by detecting fetal hypoxia early. It was accepted by obstetricians quite enthusiastically as it allowed continuous monitoring of fetal heart rate and contractions. But the studies conducted later showed that continuous electronic fetal heart rate monitoring did not significantly reduce hypoxic ischemic encephalopathy (HIE) and cerebral palsy, but it significantly increased caesarean sections and instrumental deliveries. The positive predictive value of abnormal CTG for intrapartum hypoxia is only 30% and the false positive rate is 60%. The reason is existing classification of CTG uses "pattern recognition," and this has high intra- and interobserver variability, and many patterns, like decelerations, are nonspecific. All cases of HIE are also not due to intrapartum hypoxia **(Table 1)**. So, there is a need for a paradigm shift in the classification of CTG traces. A more physiological approach to interpreting and classifying CTG traces will improve outcomes and reduce unnecessary interventions.

The first international consensus guideline on the physiological interpretation of CTG came in 2018. This is based on different types of fetal hypoxia and the fetal response to them in the CTG trace. The studies have shown that implementation of this approach has resulted in a drastic reduction in HIE in many centers. The first revision of this guideline happened in 2024, incorporating more scientific evidence, adding features of chorioamnionitis and relative uteroplacental insufficiency of labor to the interpretation table.

It is important to differentiate the normal fetal response in the CTG trace from the features of decompensation to reduce the false positive rate and unnecessary intervention. In the beginning itself, it is important to determine whether THIS fetus is "fit" to undertake the progressively hypoxic journey of labor and during labor assess the status of central oxygenation and type of hypoxia by use of "Intrapartum Fetal Assessment Tool" (How is THIS fetus?).

The basic features of CTG are baseline heart rate, baseline variability, accelerations, decelerations, and contractions.

TABLE 1: Intrapartum CTG classification.

Type of hypoxia	*Features*	*Management*
No Hypoxia	• Baseline appropriate for GA and stable • Normal variability • Presence of Cycling • No repetitive decelerations	
Chronic hypoxia	• Higher baseline than expected for GA • Reduced variability and/or absence of cycling • Absence of accelerations • Shallow decelerations	• Avoid further hypoxic stress—consider tocolysis if delay in delivery • Expedite delivery if birth is not imminent
RUPI-L (Relative uteroplacental insufficiency of labor)	• A sudden increase in FHR immediately after established contractions/induction of labor • Zigzag pattern • Widening/deepening of decelerations	Consider the overall clinical context to determine if birth should be expedited
Evolving hypoxia: Compensated	• Commonest in labor • Rise in the baseline (with normal variability and stable baseline) preceded by decelerations and loss of accelerations, with an interdeceleration interval greater than the time spent during decelerations	• Likely to respond to conservative measures • Regular review • Consider the wider clinical context
Evolving hypoxia: Decompensated	• Reduced or increased variability (Zigzag pattern), preceded by repetitive decelerations and an increase in the baseline FHR. • Unstable/progressive decline in the baseline FHR (step ladder pattern to death)	• Needs immediate intervention to reverse hypoxic stress (remove prostaglandin pessary, stop oxytocin, and/or administer tocolytic) • Delivery to be expedited if no sign of improvement
Sub-acute hypoxia	• More time in deceleration than at the baseline • Zigzag pattern	• First stage—remove PG, stop oxytocin. If there is no improvement in 10–15 mts, expedite delivery if appropriate after reviewing the overall clinical picture. • Second stage—Stop oxytocin, stop maternal

Contd...

Contd...

Type of hypoxia	*Features*	*Management*
		active pushing, if no improvement – tocolysis if delivery not imminent or expedite delivery by operative vaginal delivery
Acute hypoxia	Prolonged deceleration >3 mts	Exclude the 3 intrapartum irreversible accidents (i.e., umbilical cord prolapses, placental abruption, uterine rupture If such an accident is suspected, prepare for immediate delivery. Correct the reversible causes (uterine hyperstimulation/ hypertonus, maternal hypotension and sustained umbilical cord compression) 3-minute rule
Chorioamnionitis (SOFI)	• >10 % increase in the baseline FHR without any repetitive preceding decelerations • Loss of cycling • Zigzag or sinusoidal pattern	Consider the overall clinical context, including parity and the stage of labor, and the rate of progress of labor. In the presence of features of neuroinflammation, expedite birth to avoid the detrimental effects of superimposed hypoxia on the background fetal systemic inflammatory response syndrome (FIRS)
Other Abnormal CTG Patterns (Double Mountain Peak Sign, Poole Shark Teeth Pattern, Typical Sinusoidal Pattern, uncertain or unstable baseline)		• Exclude erroneous recording of maternal heart rate • Fetomaternal hemorrhage • Chronic fetal anemia • Fetal cardiac arrhythmias or heart blocks

BASELINE HEART RATE

The baseline heart rate reflects the myocardial function. An unstable or “wavy” baseline is an ominous feature suggestive of negative myocardial energy balance. A normal fetus should be able to maintain a gestationally age-dependent stable baseline heart rate. The normal BHR is 110–160 BPM;

for a term baby, it is 110–150 BPM. That means at 40 weeks of gestational age, BHR >150 cannot be considered normal. For preterm fetuses, we can expect values towards the upper end of this range. A sudden and abrupt drop in baseline FHR for >3 months is called prolonged deceleration. Bradycardia is BHR < 110 lasting for >10 months. Tachycardia is BHR above 160 lasting for >10 minutes. A rise in BHR by 10% of the previously observed BHR is also considered abnormal for any gestational age.

BASELINE FETAL HEART RATE VARIABILITY

The normal baseline FHRV is 5–25 BPM. The normal variability indicates a nondepressed fetal autonomic nervous system. The commonest cause of depression of the fetal autonomic nervous system is the fetal deep sleep cycle. The mean duration of deep sleep in term fetuses is approximately 15 minutes, with a maximum duration of 50 minutes in most cases. The alternate epochs of the active and quiet sleep cycle are called "fetal heart rate cycling." Cycling is a normal feature of CTG, and its absence is an ominous feature seen in the end stages of fetal hypoxia and in chorioamnionitis. The reason for the absence of cycling in chorioamnionitis is that the fetus is unable to experience deep sleep cycles due to increased neuronal metabolism. The nonphysiological causes of reduced variability are medications like opiates, end-stage hypoxia, and nonhypoxic causes like intrauterine fetal stroke. Increased variability is also important. Increased variability >25 BPM lasting >30 months is classically called "Saltatory pattern," and it is exceedingly rare in labor (5%). The more frequently seen pattern is the "Zigzag" pattern - this is an erratic fluctuation of variability >1 month and is associated with increased neonatal acidosis and requires immediate action to improve the fetal oxygenation. The zigzag pattern is seen in rapidly evolving hypoxic stress due to the injudicious use of uterotonic agents, active maternal pushing during the second stage, and in chorioamnionitis due to neuroinflammation.

ACCELERATIONS

Accelerations are considered a hallmark of a fetus in a good, oxygenated state. The fetus exposed to hypoxic stress will try to limit its body movements to conserve the available oxygen and nutrients. This leads to the absence of accelerations. But the presence of large-amplitude accelerations in labor coinciding with uterine contractions or as part of decelerations is not a true acceleration "Double Mountain Peak Sign"—may indicate erroneous recording of maternal heart rate as FHR.

DECELERATIONS

Decelerations often cause anxiety to obstetricians and lead to obstetric interventions like caesarean delivery. But decelerations are reflex cardioprotective reflexes to reduce myocardial workload when a fetus is exposed to hypoxic stress and have to be considered as a normal response. This will help to maintain aerobic metabolism in the myocardium. Actually, when there is severe hypoxia and acidosis in the fetal brain, these protective reflexes may be obliterated, leading to the absence or presence of "shallow decelerations," which are ominous compared to deep and "ugly-looking decelerations" as the latter indicate good fetal protective reflex responses to ongoing stress. Decelerations lasting more than 3 minutes are suggestive of acute hypoxia and need immediate intervention.

The traditional practice is to classify the FHR decelerations into early, variable, and late decelerations based on morphology, duration, and relation to uterine contractions. But the morphology of decelerations does not correlate with poor perinatal outcomes. The intervening baseline between ongoing decelerations must be assessed to determine its stability, presence of normal variability, and cycling. Regardless of the type of deceleration, if CTG shows a stable normal baseline and reassuring variability, then the central organs (brain, heart, and adrenals) are well oxygenated, and the risk of acidosis is low. Decelerations lasting >60 seconds, gradual recovery to baseline, persistent, and recurrent may be associated with acidosis.

It is difficult to eliminate the continuing influence of traditional obstetric teaching of classifying the decelerations based on morphology. Till the obstetricians get full confidence in physiological interpretation, the suggestion is to classify decelerations into two morphological types based on the likely underlying pathophysiological mechanisms—"Quicklie" and "Tardy."

Quicklie

Any deceleration that has an abrupt drop from the baseline (>30 BPM) and reaches the nadir in 30 seconds from the onset of deceleration and demonstrates quick recovery to the baseline. These are supposed to be due to umbilical cord compression and resultant transient hypoxemia and not due to hypoxia or acidosis. If the intervening CTG trace shows a normal baseline and variability, the oxygenation of central organs is normal. If there is an associated increase in the baseline FHR (due to catecholamine surge), then changes in the maternal position and/or reducing the rate of oxytocin may help to restore the baseline to normal.

Tardy

Any deceleration that has a gradual drop from the baseline and then recovers gradually to the baseline even after the cessation of contractions. They are due to uteroplacental insufficiency. They may be associated with acidosis if there is associated with reduced variability. Tardy decelerations are often due to structural damage to the placenta and cannot be reversed by the changes in maternal position or administration of fluids to the mother.

The "Double Mountain Peak Sign" (large amplitude accelerations coinciding with uterine contractions) is an erroneous recording of maternal heart rate. Sinusoidal pattern is a regular, smooth undulating signal resembling a sine wave with amplitude 5-15 bpm and frequency of 3-5 cycles per minute, often seen in fetomaternal hemorrhage. Atypical sinusoidal or the "Pool Shark Teeth" pattern has a more jagged saw tooth appearance rather than a smooth sine wave form, seen in acute fetal hypovolemia and hypotension.

ACUTE HYPOXIA: 3-MINUTE RULE (3,6,9,12,15 RULE)

Prolonged deceleration >3 mts in the CTG trace is suggestive of acute hypoxia. It can be due to 3 irreversible causes like abruption, cord prolapse, and uterine rupture, or 3 reversible causes like tachysystole, maternal hypotension, and umbilical cord compression. If irreversible causes are suspected, prepare for immediate delivery, and if reversible causes are suspected, correct them (3-6 mts). In suspected reversible causes, if there are no signs of recovery (improvement of variability and return of the normal baseline), in 6-9 mts preparation for immediate delivery to be started. By 9-12 mts, decelerations must have either recovered or preparation for delivery progressed, and aim for delivery by 12-15 mts. Do not follow the 3-minute rule if the deceleration is preceded by reduced variability and lack of cycling; immediate preparation should be made to expedite delivery by the safest and fastest route possible. If normal variability and cycling before and during the first 3 minutes of the deceleration are present, 90% will recover within 6 minutes and 95% in 9 minutes (if acute accidents have been excluded).

CHORIOAMNIONITIS

The fetal inflammation increases the metabolic rate and increases tissue oxygen demand, which predisposes vital organs like myocardium and neurons to hypoxic-ischemic damage. Chorioamnionitis due to ascending infection is primarily a fetal disease, and maternal signs (pyrexia and tachycardia) are late signs or may never occur in about 30% cases. Fetal Inflammatory Response Syndrome (FIRS) can cause fetal multi-organ damage. If the uterine contractions are allowed to continue, it may further reduce the oxygen supply and may potentiate the fetal compromise. The CTG features suggestive of chorioamnionitis are discussed in the interpretation table.

CONCLUSION

Despite repetitive decelerations in the CTG trace, if there is a stable baseline FHR and reassuring FHRV, then fetal acidosis is very unlikely.

SUGGESTED READING

1. Chandraharan E, Evans SA, Krueger D, et al. Physiological CTG interpretation. Intrapartum Fetal Monitoring Guideline 2018. [Online] Available from https://physiological-ctg.com/guideline.htmlhttps://physiological-ctg.com/guideline.html [Last accessed January, 2026].
2. Chandraharan E, Pereira S, Ghi T, et al. International expert consensus statement on physiological interpretation of cardiotocograph (CTG): First revision (2024). Eur J Obstet Gynecol Reprod Biol. 2024;302:346-55.

6 CHAPTER

Intrapartum Ultrasound

Chinmay Umarji, Saburi Kulkarni

INTRODUCTION

The assessment and management of patients based on clinical examination during labor has been the mainstay of traditional management. The subjective variation in clinical findings may result in an inaccurate estimation of the progress of labor and labor-related events. Intrapartum ultrasound in the form of transperineal or translabial applications for the assessment of fetal head station, position, and attitude has shown promising results in the assessment, monitoring, and documentation of labor progress. Assessment of the progress of labor by the use of intrapartum ultrasound has shown encouraging results. Reproducibility of results allows fine documentation.

INDICATIONS

- Abnormal progress of labor (slow progress/arrest).
- Before an instrumental delivery to confirm fetal head station and position.
- To diagnose or confirm a clinical diagnosis of fetal malpresentation or malposition during labor.
- Unregistered patients
- High BMI
- Suspected IUFD
- Abruptio placentae

TECHNIQUE

While performing an intrapartum ultrasound, the operator may choose to perform a transperineal or transabdominal approach depending on the indication and parameter to be assessed.

A two-dimensional *ultrasound* machine with a convex probe is used. Machines used in labor rooms should preferably have a quick start-up with rechargeable batteries.

Assessment of Fetal Head Position

Digital examinations to palpate the suture lines and fontanelles to identify the position of the fetal head have been traditionally used in obstetric practice.

It is of utmost importance to know the location of the fetal head during labor. This may be difficult in cases with the presence of caput succedaneum and asynclitism.

The convex probe is placed transversely on the maternal abdomen, and axial and sagittal planes are visualized. The position of the fetal spine is determined, and then the position of the fetal head is examined. A combination of transabdominal and transperineal ultrasound helps in better identification of fetal head position **(Table 1)**.

Assessment of Fetal Head Station

While performing a digital examination, the plane of the maternal ischial spines is the reference plane to identify the fetal head station. The descent of the head in the birth canal is assessed by examining the change in the level of the fetal head relative to the plane of the maternal ischial spine. Ultrasound helps in the assessment of the labor progress by serial examination of the fetal head station **(Table 2)**.

With an empty bladder, the patient is placed in a semirecumbent position. The ultrasound probe is placed between the two labia or further caudally at the level of the fourchette.

Quantitative measurements like the angle of progression (AoP), progression distance (PD), and the transperineal ultrasound head distance are obtained by transperineal ultrasound in the midsagittal plane. Head-to-perineum distance (HPD) is assessed in the axial plane.

ANGLE OF PROGRESSION

It is the angle formed between the long axis of the pubic bone and a line tangential to the fetal head and passing through the lowest edge of the pubic bone. It is reproducible and accurate, and helps in studying the progress of labor.

TABLE 1: Important landmarks to identify fetal head position.

Occiput and cervical spine	Occipitoanterior
Two orbits	Occipitoposterior
Midline cerebral echo	Occipito transverse

TABLE 2: Head positions depicted as a clock.

≥ 02.30 h and ≤ 03.30 h	Left occiput transverse (LOT)
≥ 08.30 h and ≤ 09.30 h	Right occiput transverse (ROT)
>03.30 h and < 08.30 h	Occiput posterior
>09.30 h and < 02.30 h	Occiput anterior

Probe Placement to Measure Angle of Progression

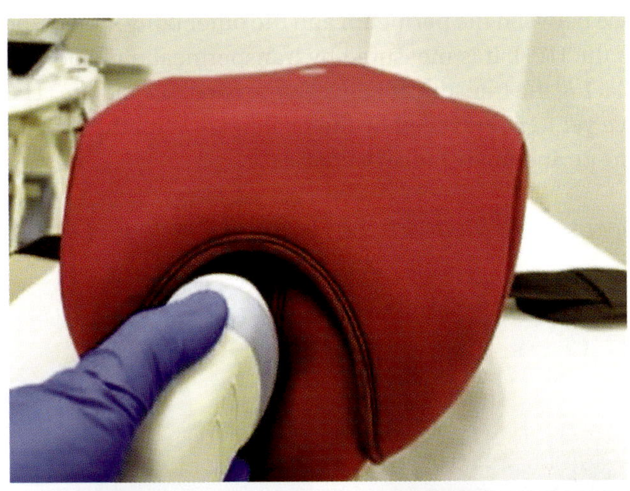

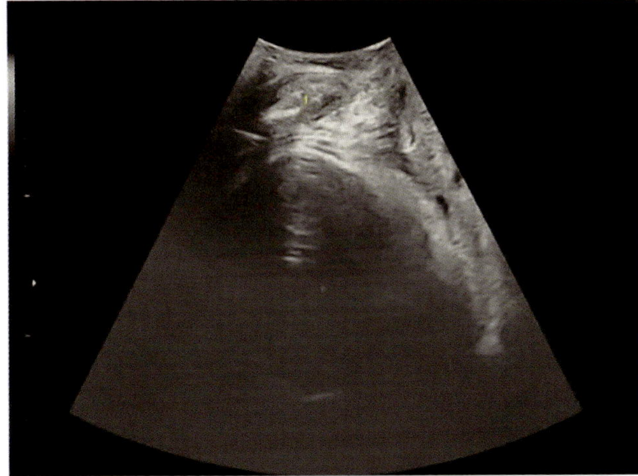

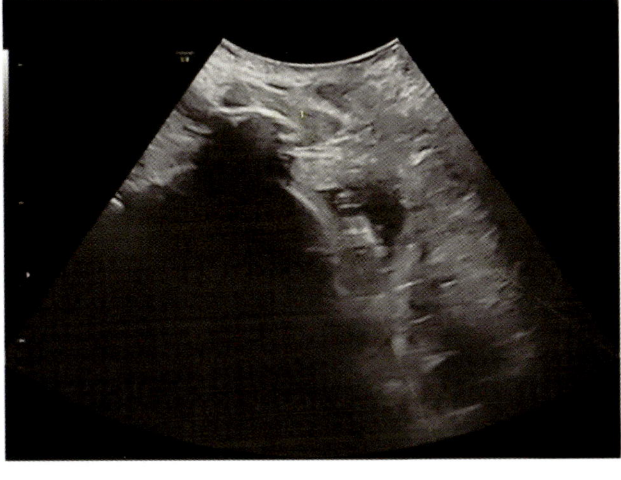

Head-to-perineum Distance

The distance between the perineum and the outer bony limit of the fetal skull is noted as the HPD. It is measured by transperineal ultrasound in the axial plane by placing the transducer between the two labia majora. This indicates the distance yet to be travelled by the fetal head. With the progress of labor, the Head-to-perineum distance decreases.

Probe Placement to Measure the Head-to-perineum Distance

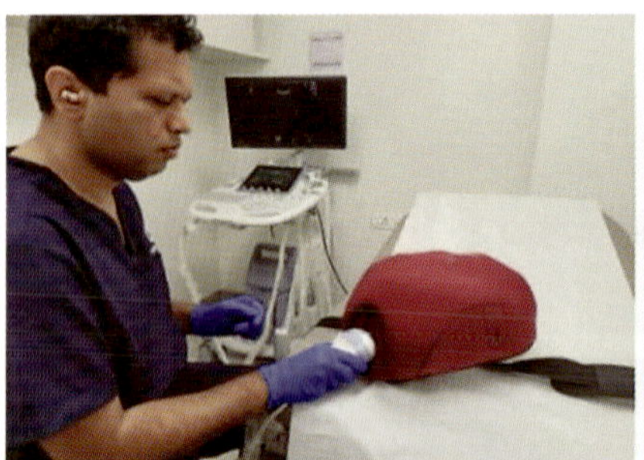

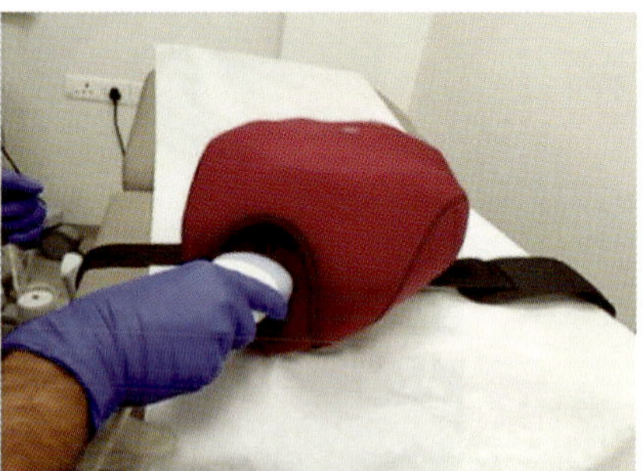

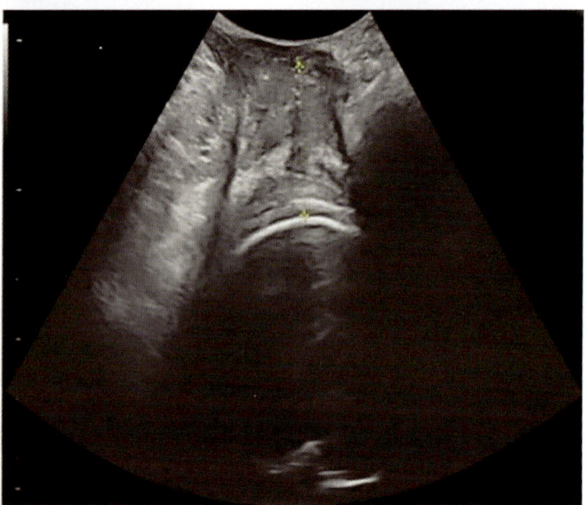

Fetal head direction: The direction of the fetal head changes with the descent of the head. Transperineal ultrasound is done in the midsagittal plane. The angle between the long axis of the pubis and the longest axis of the fetal head gives the fetal head direction.

Midline angle: The angle between the echogenic lines between the two cerebral hemispheres is called the midline angle. It is measured by transperineal ultrasound in the axial plane and helps in identifying the rotation of the fetal head as an indicator of labor progress.

Assessment of Cervical Dilatation

The ultrasound probe is held in a transverse plane at the vaginal introitus, and cervical dilatation is measured in the anteroposterior plane. There is fair agreement between the digital examination and cervical dilatation by ultrasound up to 7-8 cm, after which it is difficult to visualize the thin and effaced cervix.

PROBE PLACEMENT FOR ASSESSMENT OF CERVICAL DILATATION

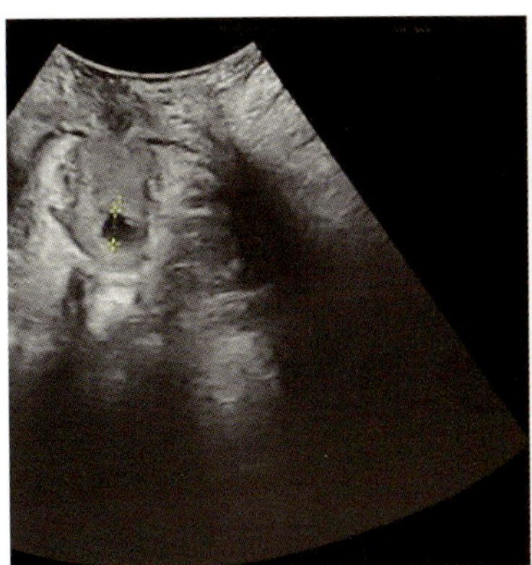

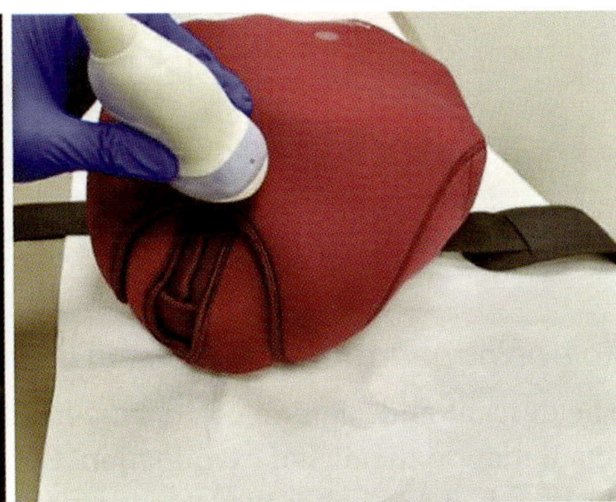

Assessment of Fetal Head Attitude

Ultrasound helps in the visualization of the fetal head attitude, which is the relationship between the fetal head and the fetal spine.

Sonopartogram

Sonopartogram is the assessment of labor based on serial ultrasound. It was introduced in 2014 and is a reproducible and complementary method to clinical assessment. With ultrasound machines being increasingly available in labor rooms, a graphical representation of labor can be obtained by entering the clinical and ultrasound results. It also serves as a fine method of documentation.

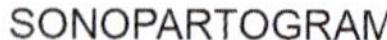

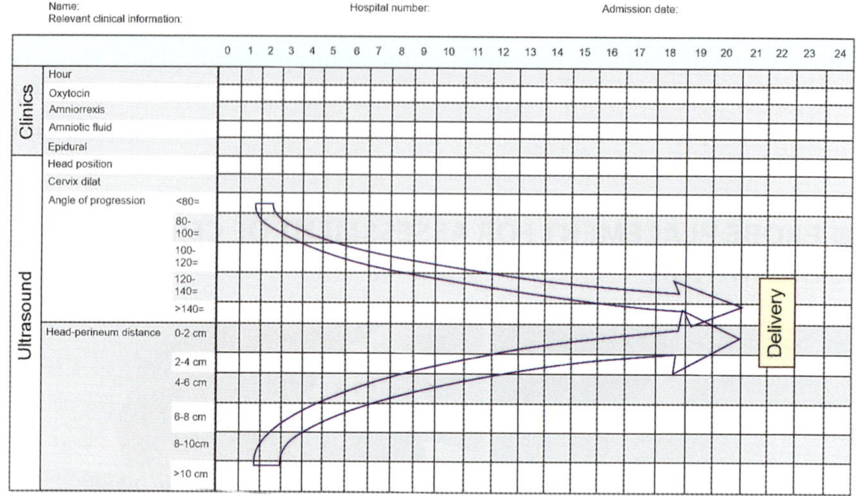

Role of Intrapartum Ultrasound in Instrumental Delivery

The descent and rotation of the fetal head can be assessed by ultrasound in addition to the digital examination. Correct knowledge of the fetal head position helps in better placement of the suction cup closer to the flexion point. The angle of progression >120 degrees helps to predict easy and successful vacuum extraction.

Documentation

Ultrasound done during labor should be noted in the indoor records. Ultrasound results for fetal viability with heart rate, fetal presentation, position, spine, and placenta should be added. As per the indication for intrapartum ultrasound, a clinician may choose to assess parameters like angle of progression (AoP), head-perineum distance (HPD), head direction with respect to pubic symphysis, and midline angle (MLA). All parameters assessed should be documented in the report.

Advantages of Intrapartum Ultrasound

- Reduce inter-observer variation due to reproducible and accurate results.
- More acceptable to patients than digital pelvic examinations.

DISADVANTAGES OF INTRAPARTUM ULTRASOUND

- Unnecessary diagnoses, e.g., Cord around the neck. One study suggested the increased risk of caesarean section in low-risk patients undergoing intrapartum ultrasound.

- Low sensitivity of ultrasound for certain conditions. E.g., Abruptio placentae
- High costs
- It is dependent on operator expertise.
- Legal (PCPNDT?)

INTRAPARTUM ULTRASOUND: SUMMARY AND CONCLUSION

- Angle of progression >120 degrees and head-to-perineum distance of less than 4 cm have excellent correlation with delivery time and probability of vaginal birth.
- Cervical dilatation is underestimated by 1-2 cm and correlates up to 7 cm dilatation. This helps to avoid repeated vaginal examinations and their discomfort and risk of infection.
- Excellent reproducibility and precise documentation.
- Patient acceptance.
- Counseling
- Evidence

The use of intrapartum ultrasound has been advised as an adjunctive method to clinical examination and not as a substitute for digital vaginal examination.

SUGGESTED READING

1. Akmal S, Kametas N, Tsoi E, et al. Comparison of transvaginal digital examination with intrapartum sonography to determine fetal head position before instrumental delivery. Ultrasound Obstet Gynecol. 2003;21(5):437-40.
2. Hassan WA, Taylor S, Lees C. Intrapartum ultrasound for assessment of cervical dilatation. Am J Obstet Gynecol MFM. 2021;3(6S):100448.
3. Usman. The sonopartogram. Am J Obstet Gynecol 2023.

7 CHAPTER

Mastering Difficult Cesarean Section

Mausumi De Banerjee, Jyoti Ramesh Chandran

INTRODUCTION

Caesarean Section is the most common operative procedure in obstetric practice but still the obstetricians face numerous challenges in managing the difficult cesarean sections.

Factors contributing to these difficulties include prior surgeries, obesity, maternal condition, fetal presentation , multiple pregnancies, placenta previa, excessive bleeding, bladder injury, fetal injury, etc.

Managing these complications requires specific surgical techniques to ensure the safety of both the mother and baby.

CAUSES OF A DIFFICULT CESAREAN SECTION

Difficult Abdominal Access

- *Types of abdominal incision:*
    - *Pfannenstiel (Bikini incision):* Most commonly used low transverse curved cut just above the pubic hair line. It is cosmetically appealing.
    - *Joel-Cohen:* Straight transverse cut 3 cm below the line connecting two superior iliac spines. It involves minimal incision through skin and subcutaneous tissue with fascia and abdominal wall bluntly opened with the fingers .It has less blood loss and shorter OT time.
    - *Maylard:* The incision extends laterally to the iliac spines and involves cutting of the rectus sheath and muscles for better exposure, especially when we suspect dense adhesions. We must be cautious of injury of the inferior epigastric arteries.
    - *Midline vertical (Classical):* In emergency for quicker access to the uterus and faster delivery of the baby. Indications are (A) Transverse lie with spontaneous rupture of membrane, (B) structural abnormality of the uterus, (C) constriction ring with neglected labor, (D) very preterm fetus with malpresentation, (E) central placenta praevia, (F) huge fibroid in the lower segment, (G) cancer cervix, (H) peri-mortem CS (to save the baby).

  There is high risk of incisional hernia, and the scar is not aesthetically pleasant.

- *Previous cesarean section:* Scar should be excised with elliptical incision, and the sides should be aligned properly.
  Peritoneum should be opened as high as possible to prevent bladder and bowel injuries

Difficult Access to the Lower Uterine Segment

Prior multiple surgeries leading to adhesions specially in previous classical Cesarean section, poorly formed or thick lower uterine segment (LUS), anterior placenta, leiomyomas, and uterine anomalies

- *Adhesiolysis:* It is done with points of scissors directed towards the uterus.
  Fibrous bands are cut carefully. Vascular omental adhesions are cut between sutures.
  Omentum must be placed between uterus and anterior abdominal wall to prevent future adhesions.
- *Uterine anomalies,* e.g., Bicornuate or didelphys—both the horns must be recognized to carefully prevent the lateral extension of the uterine incision.
  Uterine cavities should be properly cleaned to prevent PPH from placental bits.
  Sometimes the lower uterine segment is small and remains thick. So, U-, J-, or inverted T-shaped incisions are given on the uterus to prevent lateral extension. In inverted T there is more chance of intra-operative blood loss and chances of uterine rupture in future trial of labor.
- *Bladder injury:* Incidence is 0.08–0.94%.
  Incision given 2 cm above the bladder attachment and the Utero Vesicle fold is mobilized with a finger swab.
  Bladder injury happens while (i) creation of the bladder flap—43%; (ii) entry to peritoneum-33%, (iii) during uterine incision and delivery of the baby—24%
  95% dome of the bladder is injured and rest is the trigone.
  Repair done in two layers by 3-0 absorbable sutures. First layer simple running, second layer continuous interlocking. Catheter kept in situ for 10 days approximately.
- *Leiomyomas:* 0.3–7.2% cases.
  Cesarean myomectomy done, if very big fibroid in lower segment-classical CS is performed.
- *Anterior low-lying placenta:* Fingers are insinuated in an area free of placenta, or transplacental access is used if the placenta fully covers the entry
  Preoperative planning and placental localization is important.

Dee Lee incision (Lower vertical) given if poorly developed or highly vascular lower segment or with high up presenting part.

Difficulty in Delivering the Fetus

Abnormal fetal presentations include:

- *Floating head:* It may happen when lower uterine segment is not formed or is highly vascular. Amniotomy is done to drain out the amniotic fluid completely, which allows the descent of the presenting part. The use of one blade of forceps as Vectis or both blades of forceps or cup of ventouse may facilitate the process to deliver the baby. Internal podalic version may be tried.
- *Deeply engaged head:* 1.5% cases.
    - *Abdominovaginal delivery:* A lot of fetal risks involved like intra-cranial hemorrhage, skull or neck fractures, asphyxia, etc.
      Mother may also suffer from uterine and cervical injuries and severe hemorrhage.
    - *Reverse breech extraction:* First delivery of the podalic end of the fetus followed by the fetal head. In this method wound extension and uterine vessel injury becomes less.
    - *Patwardhan's technique:* The uterine incision is made at the level of the shoulders of the fetus. followed by delivery of one shoulder, then the other making the back anterior (occipitoanterior) then the trunk keeping two hands on the ventral aspect of the fetus and on the buttocks along with the legs are delivered followed by the head.
    - *Fetal pillows:* Silicone balloon inflated with 180 mL sterile saline is used vaginally for elevation of the deeply engaged head. It reduces maternal and fetal morbidity.
    - *Forceps:* Single blade using as vectis or with the double blade fetus delivered through uterine wound. There is high chance of extension of uterine incision.

Malpresentation of the Fetus

Extracting the fetus in breech or transverse lie often requires grasping a limb for gentle extraction; poorly executed maneuvers can result in nerve injury or bone fracture

If the second twin is larger or in transverse lie or in viable conjoined twin cesarean section to be performed very carefully.

In cord presentation, if the cervix is not fully dilated the baby can be saved by quick delivery by CS.

Intraoperative Excessive Blood Loss

Call for help and resuscitation of the patient is very important with fluids, blood, oxytocics, etc.

- *Precautions to be taken to minimize blood loss during CS:*
    - Loose UV peritoneum should be incised.
    - Preoperative planning with USG localization of the fetus and the placenta is essential for appropriate incision and fetal delivery without uterine incision extension
    - Controlled cord traction with oxytocics is preferred over manual removal of placenta.
    - The angles of the uterine incision should be secured carefully.
- *PAS (Placenta accreta spectrum):* In patients with prior CS where USG shows anterior low-lying placenta, chances of morbid adherent placenta to be kept in mind. Bladder may also be involved with high risk of bladder and ureteric injuries.

    In such cases proper counseling to be done with consent for Cesarean Hysterectomy. Delivery must be planned in a tertiary care center (level III or IV) with ICU, NICU and with access to blood bank. An expert team of obstetricians, anesthetist, pediatrician and preferably urosurgeon must be available.

    Expectant management: Cord is ligated close to the placenta and left in situ. IV Methotrexate is given for involution of the placenta. It is not recommended now as there is high chances of maternal hemorrhagic, neurologic and nephrologic side effects. Follow up MRI is needed. There are chances of infection and secondary hysterectomy may be required.

    Extirpative management with forcible partial manual removal of placenta with suturing of placental bed and balloon tamponade is abandoned by FIGO 2018, due to chances of massive hemorrhage.

    Cesarean hysterectomy is the treatment of choice.
- *Intraoperative hemorrhage:* It may also be due to atonic uterus or inadvertent tears.
    - *External Aortic compression:* It is an effective method to reduce the blood loss temporarily until alternative measures are taken.
    - *Stepwise devascularization:* Ligation of vessels are as follows—Unilateral uterine vessel at the upper part of the lower uterine segment, bilateral uterine vessels, cervicovaginal branches, vaginal artery (after pushing the bladder down to avoid ureteric injuries), unilateral ovarian vessel, bilateral ovarian vessels, unilateral or bilateral ligation of internal iliac artery ligation may be necessary.
    - *Compression Sutures-B Lynch suture* was introduced by Chrsitopher B Lynch in 1997. Use of vertical brace sutures to compress the anterior and posterior walls of the uterus. It is indicated only when bimanual compression of the uterus decreases the vaginal bleeding.

Cho multiple sutures: With multiple square sutures anterior and posterior walls of the uterus are approximated leaving no space in between.

INDICATIONS OF CESAREAN HYSTERECTOMY—SUBTOTAL OR TOTAL

- Intractable uterine atony
- Uncontrolled bleeding from lower segment of uterus due to—laceration of major vessels, placental implantation, extension of uterine incision laterally causing avulsion of uterine arteries into the broad ligament or extending downwards causing colporrhexis (separation of the cervix from the vaginal fornix)
- Morbid adhesion of placenta
- Large fibroids
- Uterine rupture, which cannot be repaired
- Cornual or cervical pregnancy
- Recurrent uterine inversion

Fetal injuries may occur like scalp lacerations, skull fractures, nerve injuries (brachial plexus, spinal cord), long bone fractures, liver hematomas, perinatal asphyxia, intracranial hemorrhage, or even death

Gentle handling, avoiding hasty extraction, and mastery of maneuvers are very important.

CONCLUSION

Anticipating complications and preoperative planning of CS based on maternal anatomy, fetal presentation, placental location with proficiency in evidence-based maneuvers are essential for minimizing the risks and improving outcomes for both mother and baby.

SUGGESTED READING

1. Alves ÁLL, Nozaki AM, da Silva LB. Difficult fetal extraction in cesarean section: Number 8 - 2024. Rev Bras Ginecol Obstet. 2024;46:e-FPS08.
2. Dalvi SA. Difficult Deliveries in Cesarean Section. J Obstet Gynaecol India. 2018;68(5):344-8.
3. Harmony EL. J Obgy. 2005;25(2):143-9.
4. Shobhana. Systemic Stepwise devascularization. TOGS. 2006;2(3).
5. Visconti F, Quaresima P, Rania E, et al. Difficult caesarean section: A literature review. Eur J Obstet Gynecol Reprod Biol. 2020;246:72-8.

8 CHAPTER

Maternal Collapse in Labor Room

Jyotsna Suri

INTRODUCTION

Maternal collapse is a life-threatening emergency which may occur even in women without any high-risk factors. It may occur in the antenatal period, during labor or in the postpartum period. It is defined as an acute event involving the cardiorespiratory and or the central nervous system leading to reduced or absent conscious level and potentially cardiac arrest and death in any stage of pregnancy and up to 6 weeks in the post-partum period. The reported incidence of this condition is about 1 per 16,000 maternities with a survival rate of 58%.

WHAT ARE THE CAUSES OF MATERNAL COLLAPSE?

Maternal collapse can be due to pregnancy related or unrelated to pregnancy causes. Common causes of collapse are bleeding during pregnancy or after delivery, high blood pressure leading to complications like stoke and convulsions (eclampsia), sepsis and rarely drug reactions or anesthesia complications.

The causes of maternal collapse in most situations are reversible and hence the need for alacrity in the response to maternal collapse. There are some mnemonics which help us to remember the causes of maternal collapse. The first one is the ABCDEFGH, where A—Anesthesia complications, B—Bleeding, C—Cardiac, D—Drugs, E—Embolism, F—Fever (sepsis), G—general (electrolyte imbalance, hypoxia), H—Hypertension.

Another way to remember is the 4H and 4T. The 4 H—hypovolemia, hypoxia, hypo-hyperkalemia, and hypo-hyperthermia; the 4 Ts are: Thromboembolism, Toxicity (drug), Tension (pneumothorax), and tamponade (cardiac).

CAN MATERNAL COLLAPSE BE PREDICTED?

Sometimes high-risk pregnancies like preeclampsia, multiple pregnancies, repeated cesarean sections and severe anemia can have complications. During labor if they are carefully monitored using obstetric early warning scores, timely action can be taken. However very often a normal patient with no high-risk factors can collapse without any warning signs.

WHAT IS THE ROLE OF HEALTH CARE PROVIDER WHEN THEY FACE SUCH A SITUATION?

Besides providing medical care the role of communication and counseling of the near and dear ones is of utmost importance. The details of the condition should be periodically informed in simple language and all treatment options explained.

HOW IS MATERNAL COLLAPSE TREATED?

The initial response is to resuscitate the patient using the C-A-B protocol of basic life support (BLS). After patient is stabilized the definite reason for collapse is determined and targeted treatment is instituted.

Initial Response for Maternal Collapse

- CALL FOR HELP—Call the senior obstetrician, anesthesiologist, neonatologist, nursing staffs and extra residents immediately.
- Assess ABCDE simultaneously as well as responsiveness by AVPU scale. Feel for the carotid pulse for not more than 10 seconds. If carotid is absent start straight away with good quality compressions.
- Begin early high-quality CPR—C-A-B-D
- Airway patency can be assessed by whether patient is vocalizing and by any loud gurgling sounds indicating compromised airway.
- Breathing is assessed by respiratory rate and SpO_2. Oxygen by mask is started at 6-8 L/min.
- Circulation is assessed by blood pressure. Two wide bore canula (18 or 16 G should be secured) above the diaphragm
- Displace gravid uterus-manually, (left uterine displacement).
- Minimum 4 BLS responders for effective CPR

FEATURES OF GOOD QUALITY COMPRESSIONS

- Rate of CPR should be 100–120/min and ratio of compressions to ventilation is 30:2.
- Compression should be given at the lower half of the sternum between the nipples with heel of one hand and the other hand on top with fingers interlocked
- Push chest hard and fast. It should be compressed at least by 5–6 cm.
- Allow complete recoil of the chest wall
- Do not bend your elbows when doing chest compressions; doing so will deliver weak, ineffective chest compression.
- The time interval between each compression and relaxation should be approximately the same
- Minimize any interruptions to chest compression (hands-off time)

- If available, use a prompt and/or feedback device to help ensure high quality chest compressions.
- Do not rely on palpating carotid or femoral pulses to assess the effectiveness of chest compressions.
- Resume compressions without any delay; place your hands back on the center of the patient's chest (lower part of sternum)

OTHER COMPONENTS OF RESUSCITATION

Use a bag and mask to start ventilation and supplemental oxygen should be added as soon as possible. A tight seal should be formed over the nose and with one hand such that a "C" and "E" is formed. The other hand should be used to inflate the bag **(Fig. 1)**. The inspiratory time should be around 1 second. Give enough volume to produce a visible rise of the chest wall. Avoid rapid or forceful breaths.

- As soon as a defibrillator is available, the self-adhesive pads should be applied to the chest. Do not interrupt compressions during this process. The heart rhythm will be assessed with the electrodes during a brief pause (less than 5 seconds) in compressions.
- If the rhythm is ventricular fibrillation/pulseless ventricular tachycardia (VF/pVT), start defibrillation. The energy used is the same as for nonpregnant patients.
- Restart chest compressions immediately. Do not delay restarting chest compressions to check the cardiac rhythm.
- If rhythm is nonshockable—asystole or pulseless electrical activity, do not defibrillate but continue CPR

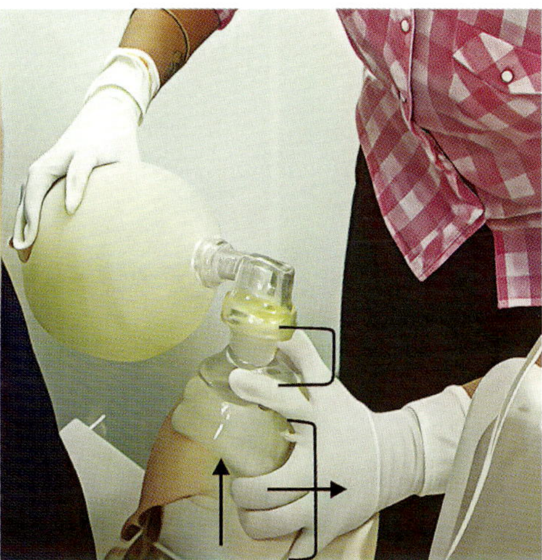

Fig. 1: Technique of bag and mask ventilation; C—compresses the bag for a tight seal on the face; E—elevates the jaw.

- If there is no access, IV access should be established once resuscitation is underway so as to deliver the drugs. Injection adrenaline 1 mg IV, every 3–5 minutes, if non shockable rhythm; In case of refractory ventricular fibrillation, injection amiodarone, 300 mg IV

HOW IS RESUSCITATION DIFFERENT IN A PREGNANT WOMAN?

Chest compressions are performed in the same way as in a non-pregnant person EXCEPT that if the pregnant uterus is above the umbilicus, it should be tilted towards the left side with one hand or both hands by the assisting personnel (LUD) **(Figs. 2A and B)**. The perimortem cesarean also called resuscitative hysterotomy is also a component of maternal resuscitation if the pregnant uterus is above the umbilicus.

If CPR is not effective, consider resuscitative hysterotomy (also called perimortem cesarean delivery):

- PMCD should be considered at 4 minutes after onset of maternal cardiac arrest or resuscitative efforts (for the un-witnessed arrest) if there is no maternal ROSC—AHA 2015 Guidelines
- In patients who are > 20 weeks of pregnancy. Before 20 weeks of gestation there is no proven benefit from delivery of the fetus and placenta. Perimortem caesarean section should be considered a resuscitative procedure to be performed primarily in the interests of maternal, not fetal, survival

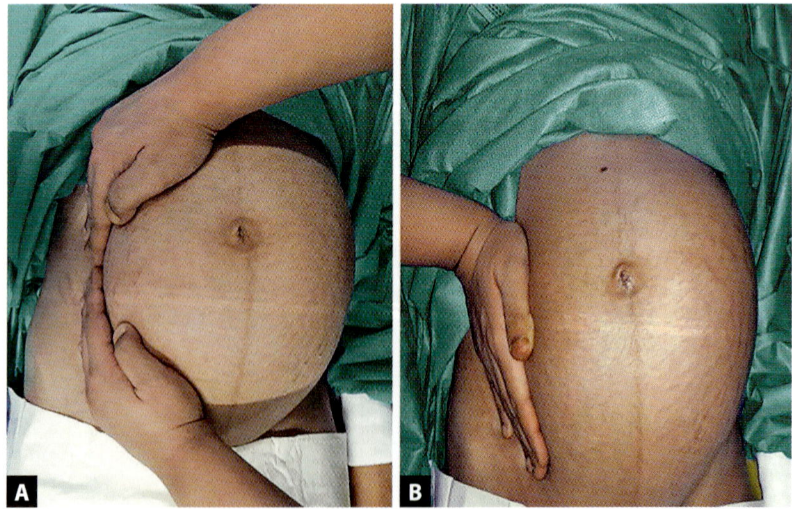

Figs. 2A and B: One-handed and two-handed method to achieve left uterine displacement (LUD).

DEFINITIVE MANAGEMENT OF MATERNAL COLLAPSE

Targeted History

- History of past illness(anemia and heart disease), past pregnancies, previous surgeries
- History of present pregnancy-hypertension, anemia, breathlessness, antepartum hemorrhage, leaking, fever, excessive vomiting, and headache
- History of labor and delivery
- Drug history/anesthetics
- History of third stage
- Think of 4 H (hypovolemia, hypoxia, Hyper/hypokalemia, and hypothermia) and 4 T (thrombosis, tamponade, toxins, and tension pneumothorax)

General Examination

- Assess sensorium by AVPU scale
- Skin/mucous membrane—pallor and sweating
- Neck veins are normal or full
- Pulse/Respiration/Temperature
- Generalized anasarca, pedal edema
- Blood pressure
- Heart—any murmurs
- Lung—breath sounds, crepitations, and rhonchi
- Abdominal examination—uterine size, contractility, tenderness
- Local vulva—ongoing bleeding, clots
- Per speculum and vaginal examination—cervical/vaginal lacerations, hematoma

Investigations

- Basic investigations—CBC, LKT/KFT, coagulation profile, serum electrolytes, blood glucose, and urine routine
- Blood group and cross match
- Pulse oximetry, ECG, and cardiac monitoring,
- Arterial blood gases
- Portable chest X-ray
- Point-of-care ultrasound (POCUS)

Based on the targeted history and examination and the POCUS and other investigations the targeted management is administered. Some important causes of non-hemorrhagic collapse and the management principles are shown in **Table 1**.

TABLE 1: Important causes of nonhemorrhagic maternal collapse and management principles.

Condition	*Specific Management*
Anaphylaxis	Anaphylaxis: 1:1,000 adrenaline 500 micrograms (0.5 mL) intramuscularly
$MgSO_4$ toxicity	10 mL of 10% calcium gluconate IV, slow
Sepsis	1-hour sepsis bundle
Eclampsia	$MgSO_4$, blood pressure control, supportive care
Pulmonary embolism	Heparin/LMWH, supportive care
Uterine inversion	Manual reposition
Cardiac failure	Inotropes, diuretics, and ventilation
AFE (amniotic fluid embolism)	Supportive care, FFP, and cryoprecipitate
CVA (cerebrovascular accident)	Multidisciplinary management

MANAGEMENT OF COMMON CAUSES OF MATERNAL COLLAPSE—NONHEMORRHAGIC

See **Table 1**.

KEY POINTS

- Any pregnancy can become high risk with severe outcomes
- Obstetricians should be trained to recognize maternal collapse promptly and initiate resuscitative measures
- In case of maternal cardiac arrest perimortem cs section improves outcomes if performed in 4–5 minutes
- Remember the physiological changes in pregnancy while resuscitation. LUD of uterus is imperative for effective CPR
- It is very important to have regular drills of CPR for maternal collapse for all doctors so that no mistakes are made.

SUGGESTED READING

1. Beckett VA, Knight M, Sharpe P. The CAPS Study: incidence, management and outcomes of cardiac arrest in pregnancy in the UK: a prospective, descriptive study. BJOG. 2017;124(9):1374-81.
2. Del Rios M, Bartos JA, Panchal AR, et al. Part 1: Executive Summary: 2025 American Heart Association Guidelines for Cardiopulmonary Resuscitation and Emergency Cardiovascular Care. Circulation. 2025;152(16_suppl_2): S284-S312.

9 CHAPTER

Management of Postpartum Hemorrhage in Labor Room: Protocols and Practical Approach

Sheela V Mane

INTRODUCTION

Postpartum hemorrhage (PPH) is a leading cause of maternal morbidity and mortality and requires prompt recognition and immediate management in the labor room. Effective management depends on early assessment, simultaneous resuscitation, and timely treatment directed at the underlying cause. The common causes of PPH can be broadly grouped into uterine atony, genital tract trauma, retained placental tissue, and coagulation disorders.

Primary PPH refers to blood loss of 500 mL or more from the genital tract within 24 hours of childbirth. It is further classified as minor (500–1,000 mL) and major (>1,000 mL), with major PPH subdivided into moderate (1,001–2000 mL) and severe (>2,000 mL). In women with low body weight, smaller volumes of blood loss may still be clinically significant. Secondary PPH is defined as excessive vaginal bleeding occurring from 24 hours up to 12 weeks after delivery.

PROTOCOLS AND PRACTICAL APPROACH

All delivery units should be prepared to manage postpartum hemorrhage, as it may occur even in women without known risk factors. Management requires a coordinated approach with simultaneous resuscitation, close monitoring, appropriate investigations, and prompt measures to control bleeding.

Assessment should include evaluation for hypovolemia. Physiological expansion of blood volume during pregnancy can delay the appearance of shock. Vital signs often remain within normal limits until blood loss exceeds 1,000 mL. Blood loss of 1,000–1,500 mL may be associated with tachycardia, tachypnoea, and a mild fall in systolic blood pressure. A systolic blood pressure <80 mm Hg, along with marked tachycardia, tachypnoea, and altered sensorium, usually reflects severe hemorrhage exceeding 1,500 mL.

Uterine atony is the most common cause of primary postpartum hemorrhage. Uterotonic drugs are the first-line treatment in such cases. These agents promote uterine contraction, facilitating placental separation before delivery and compressing uterine blood vessels after placental expulsion, thereby reducing bleeding. When bleeding persists, more than one uterotonic agent may be required, administered sequentially to achieve effective uterine contraction.

The following measures should be carried out sequentially to control bleeding. The uterus should be assessed and bimanual uterine massage performed to stimulate contractions. The bladder must be emptied using a Foley catheter, which should be left in situ. Oxytocin 5 IU should be administered by slow intravenous injection and may be repeated if required. Ergometrine 0.5 mg may be given intramuscularly or slowly intravenously, except in women with hypertension. An oxytocin infusion of 40 IU diluted in 500 mL of isotonic crystalloid may be commenced at a rate of 125 mL/h, unless fluid restriction is indicated. Carboprost 0.25 mg may be administered intramuscularly at intervals of at least 15 minutes, up to a maximum of eight doses, with caution in women with asthma. Misoprostol 800 µg may be given via the sublingual route. Injection tranexamic acid 1 g intravenously is also an effective alternative.

Oxytocin is the preferred first-line uterotonic for both prevention and treatment of postpartum hemorrhage. It acts by stimulating uterine smooth muscle contraction through binding to myometrial receptors. The drug can be administered intravenously or intramuscularly and has a rapid onset of action. Excessive doses or prolonged infusion may lead to fluid retention and hyponatremia, presenting with symptoms such as headache, nausea, drowsiness, or seizures. The characteristics of commonly used uterotonic agents are summarized in **Table 1**.

Immediate resuscitation should begin with warmed isotonic crystalloid fluids. Oxygen therapy should be administered to maintain oxygen saturation above 95% during initial stabilization.

Early laboratory evaluation is essential. Where laboratory facilities are limited, bedside clotting assessment may be used as a screening tool. Prolonged clotting time suggests depletion of coagulation factors and indicates the need for blood component therapy. Standard investigations should include blood grouping and cross-matching, complete blood count, coagulation profile with fibrinogen levels, and serum electrolytes. During massive transfusion, ionized calcium and potassium levels may become abnormal and require regular monitoring.

When bleeding persists despite medical management, surgical intervention should not be delayed and must be undertaken promptly based on the clinical situation.

MINIMALLY INVASIVE INTERVENTIONS

Uterine Tamponade

When bleeding continues despite medical treatment and exclusion of correctable causes, uterine tamponade may be effective, particularly in

TABLE 1: Commonly used uterotonic agents in the management of postpartum hemorrhage.

Drug	*Usual dose*	*Route of administration*	*Dosing pattern*	*Onset of action (min)*	*Common adverse effects*	*Major contraindications*
Oxytocin	10–40 IU diluted in crystalloid solution	IV infusion, IV bolus*, IM	Continuous or repeat dosing	1–5	Nausea, vomiting, hypotension, fluid retention	None
Misoprostol	200–1,000 µg	Sublingual, oral, rectal	Single administration	30–60	Fever, chills, diarrhea, nausea	None
Methylergometrine	200 µg	IM, IV*, oral	Every 2–4 hours	2–5	Hypertension, nausea, vomiting	Hypertension, migraine, peripheral vascular disease
Carboprost ($PGF_{2\alpha}$)	250 µg	IM, intramyometrial	Every 15–20 min (maximum 8 doses)	15–30	Diarrhea, vomiting, flushing, fever	Asthma, cardiac, renal or hepatic disease
Dinoprostone ($PGF_{2\alpha}$)	20 mg	Rectal	Every 2 hours	~10	Fever, chills, headache, diarrhea	Hypotension

*IV bolus administration should be slow and under close monitoring.
(IM: intramuscular; IV: intravenous; IU: intrauterine; PG: prostaglandin)

cases of uterine atony. Tamponade can be achieved using gauze packing, intrauterine balloon devices such as a Bakri or Foley catheter, or suction-based systems. Intrauterine balloon tamponade is considered an appropriate first-line procedural intervention when atony is the primary cause of hemorrhage.

Uterine Artery Embolization

In hemodynamically stable patients with access to interventional radiology, uterine artery embolization may be used to control ongoing bleeding. The technique involves selective occlusion of the uterine arteries or the anterior division of the internal iliac arteries using embolic materials, thereby reducing uterine blood flow. High success rates have been reported with this approach in appropriately selected cases.

Aortic Compression

Temporary reduction of pelvic blood flow may be used as a bridge to definitive treatment in severe postpartum hemorrhage. Resuscitative endovascular balloon occlusion of the aorta (REBOA) involves percutaneous placement of a balloon catheter under imaging guidance, with inflation above the iliac bifurcation. This technique has been successfully used in obstetric hemorrhage and as an adjunct during management of placenta accreta spectrum disorders.

Conservative surgical options may be attempted as second-line measures, depending on the clinical situation and availability of expertise.

SURGICAL INTERVENTIONS

Exploratory laparotomy is indicated when bleeding persists despite minimally invasive measures. Surgical management initially aims to reduce blood flow to the uterus and pelvis and to control the bleeding source. Definitive surgery may be required if conservative measures fail.

Artery Ligation

Bilateral uterine artery ligation is performed by identifying the uterine arteries at the level of the lower uterine segment and securing them with sutures that include the surrounding myometrium. If bleeding continues, stepwise devascularization may be extended to include additional uterine branches or the utero-ovarian pedicles.

Uterine Compression Sutures

Uterine compression sutures are used to mechanically compress the uterus and control atonic bleeding. An absorbable suture is placed through the lower uterine segment and looped over the fundus to achieve sustained compression. Several modifications of this technique have been described, with comparable effectiveness.

Hysterectomy

Hysterectomy remains the definitive treatment for postpartum hemorrhage unresponsive to all other interventions, particularly in cases of placenta accreta spectrum or uterine rupture. The decision should be made without delay when indicated. Whenever possible, involvement of a second experienced obstetrician is advisable before proceeding.

SUGGESTED READING

1. American College of Obstetricians and Gynecologists. Practice Bulletin No. 183: Postpartum hemorrhage. Obstet Gynecol. 2017;130(4):e168-86.
2. B-Lynch C, Coker A, Lawal AH, et al. The B-Lynch surgical technique for the control of massive postpartum hemorrhage: an alternative to hysterectomy? Br J Obstet Gynaecol. 1997;104(3):372-5.
3. Shakur H, Roberts I, Fawole B, et al. Effect of early tranexamic acid administration on mortality, hysterectomy, and other morbidities in women with postpartum haemorrhage (WOMAN trial). Lancet. 2017;389(10084):2105-16.
4. World Health Organization. WHO recommendations for the prevention and treatment of postpartum haemorrhage. Geneva: World Health Organization; 2012.

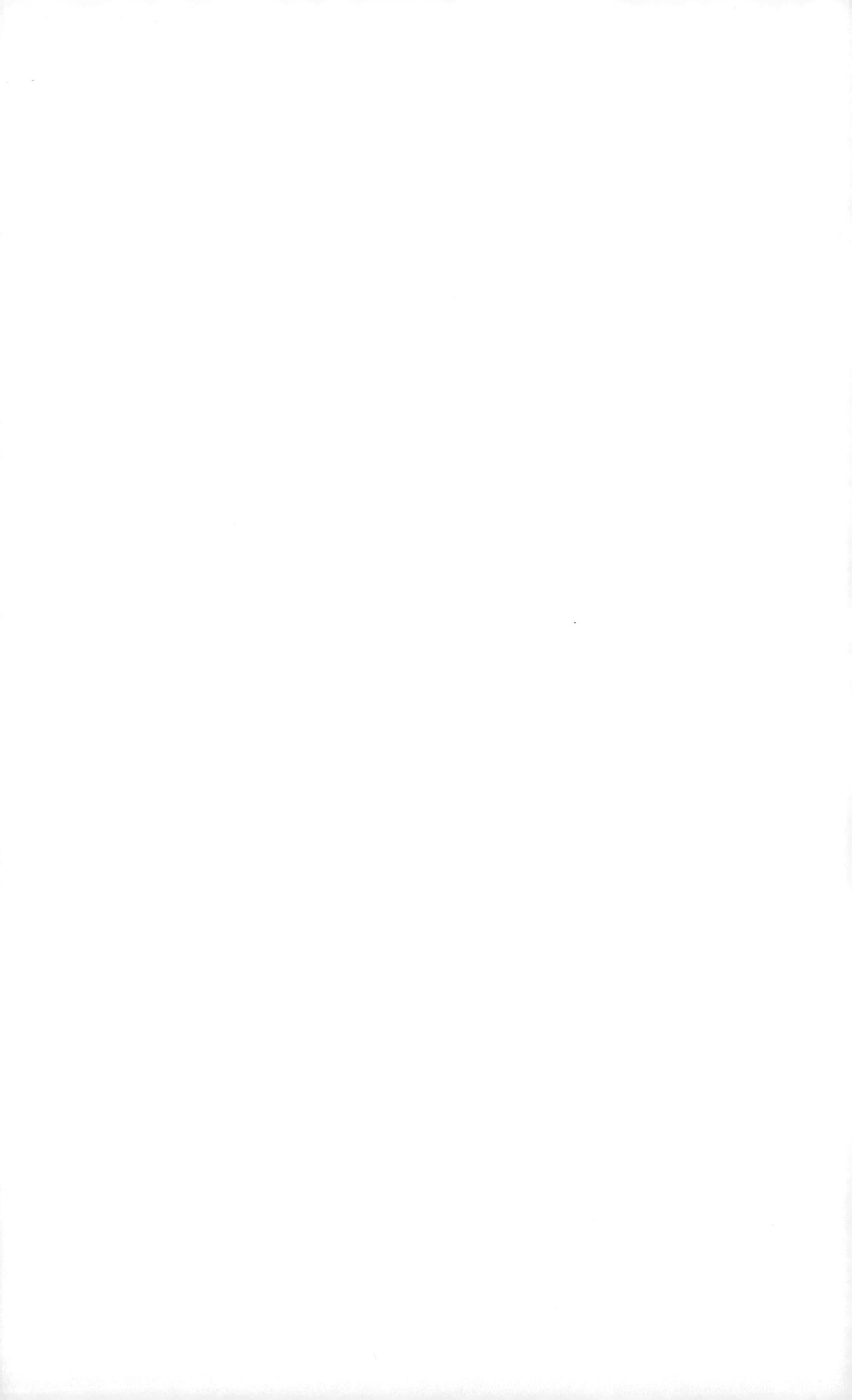